ULTIMATE OBSTACLE
RACE TRAINING

CRUSH THE WORLD'S TOUGHEST COURSES

BRETT STEWART

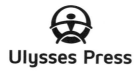

Ulysses Press

This book is dedicated to my big brother Chad. Surviving your wedgies, noogies, and "blindside QB hits" instilled the desire in me to repeatedly get back up, dust off, and ask for more. Thank you for the "torture"—I loved every second of it!

Published in the United States by
Ulysses Press
P.O. Box 3440
Berkeley, CA 94703
www.ulyssespress.com

ISBN13: 978-1-61243-104-8
Library of Congress Control Number 2012940426

Printed in the United States by Bang Printing

10 9 8 7 6 5 4 3 2 1

Acquisitions Editor: Keith Riegert
Managing Editor: Claire Chun
Editor: Lily Chou
Proofreader: Lauren Harrison
Indexer: Sayre Van Young
Cover design: what!design @ whatweb.com
Cover photographs: © Mac Stone/Savage Race
Interior photographs: see page 148
Models: Michael Bennett, Brian Burns, Tricia Burns, Evan Clontz, Lewis Elliot, Vincent Fountain, Lauren Harrison, Joseph Nusairat, Brett Stewart, Kristen Stewart, Jennifer Zoberg

Distributed by Publishers Group West

PLEASE NOTE: This book has been written and published strictly for informational purposes, and in no way should be used as a substitute for consultation with health care professionals. You should not consider educational material herein to be the practice of medicine or to replace consultation with a physician or other medical practitioner. The author and publisher are providing you with information in this work so that you can have the knowledge and can choose, at your own risk, to act on that knowledge. The author and publisher also urge all readers to be aware of their health status and to consult health care professionals before beginning any health program.

Contents

PART 1: OVERVIEW

Introduction

"We send people into death, and then we bring them back. I'm a provider. A provider of fear. For those who want it—if you're mentally tough, you can stand up against the world."
—Billy Wilson (a.k.a. Mr. Mouse), founder, Tough Guy

Our lives are filled with challenges we must endure, barriers we must navigate, and obstacles we must overcome. From the moment we learn to crawl as infants, so starts the process of developing the skills, strength, and tenacity to control the path we travel and choose our own destiny.

By the time we've "grown up" (whatever that actually means), it seems that our race against time, with countless pitfalls and potholes in our way, has become second nature. A ho-hum ordinary existence can be summed up in the following dialog between two friends over a beer:

"Hey bud, what's up?"

"Same-old, same-old. You?"

"Yup, me, too. Pass the nuts, will ya?"

A select few have drawn a line in the sand and stand together to oppose monotony, mediocrity, and lame conversation while passing a bowl of beer nuts. These renegades can be found in all walks of life, from your coffee barista sporting a neck tattoo, to the police officer who let you off with a warning for going just a wee bit over the speed limit, to your neighborhood postman who seems to relish the occasional chase by a wayward pooch. They're all around us, and most likely look just like you and me. These driven individuals have found the razor-thin line that separates the daily tasks we need to navigate and the obstacles we seek out to tackle for fun, sport, and the pure challenge of pushing our minds and bodies to their limits. They stand together as an alliance of endorphin junkies, endurance athletes, and the passionate few that crush all the barriers in their way. They are *Obstacle Racers.*

> "What we're offering is a fun, genuinely tough experience that people can be proud of."
> —Guy Livingstone, Tough Mudder

Obstacle races and mud runs have blossomed into a relatively overnight sensation across the globe, and hundreds of thousands of participants sign up and compete in these events on a weekly basis across all seven continents. (Yes, plans are being hatched to host events even in Antarctica.) Featuring each of the elements (earth, wind, fire, and water—or more accurately mud, water, ice, fire, water-soluble paint) and obstacles ranging from simple cargo nets, climbing ropes, 950-pound tractor tires, or gladiators wielding pugil sticks, there's enough variety and adrenaline-inducing activity for anyone. Not enough? Did I mention being chased by zombies?

In just the last five years, hundreds of new events have sprouted up all across America and new mega-event companies have been created to host dozens of events per year. *Spartan Race*, for example, has grown from its inaugural event in 2009 to over 60 races held worldwide in just three years, while *Warrior Dash* celebrated its one-millionth registration in early 2012.

One thing's for sure: Events based around running, climbing, jumping, ducking, crawling, dodging, and sliding will continue their rapid ascension to the forefront of weekend warrior sporting events, and quite possibly supplant some other more-entrenched pastimes. Says Alex Patterson, CMO of *Tough Mudder*, "By the end of 2012, we aim to replace Ironman as the preeminent brand in endurance sports." Kids aren't left out of the fun, either. Many events have smaller mud runs just for children under 12, and established races such as Spartan Race have taken the initiative to expand on kid-friendly courses and make them an event unto themselves.

Obstacle racers come in all shapes, sizes, and ages. *Obstacle Race Training* is dedicated to those daring individuals seeking adventure and challenges that you just can't find in most gyms. In this book you'll find dozens of tips, tricks, and techniques for conquering obstacles of every shape and size that you'll find out on most race courses, from rope climbs to flipping huge tractor tires and all the mud-based stuff you can imagine in between. I've also created three different training programs specifically designed to match real-world courses and the challenges you'll have to overcome to get to the finish line. Need the strength and technique to climb walls, evade zombies, crawl under barbed wire without a scratch, or drag heavy blocks of concrete attached to chains? This book has you covered. The knowledge and training you'll get from this book will make you a smarter, stronger, and faster obstacle racer—you just need to provide the sweat and effort and commit to do the work to crush the world's most bad-ass courses!

How Did I Get Here?

During the research and "testing" for this book, I surely earned my diploma in mud racing by sucking it up, slathering on some sunscreen, and spending countless hours building the obstacle courses that thousands of you love to hate. I braved the Arizona sun with searing triple-digit temperatures to construct a foot-grabbing tire pit from hell alongside the founders of LoziLu Women's Mud Runs. I hung off a forklift to build a webbed monster of a cargo net with Devon and the team at Cahoots Duo Challenge. Spartan Race Gladiator Arena? Been there and swung the pugil sticks to prove it.

I was the guy inside the wrecked cars at Tough Mudder shooting photos while hundreds of you maniacs were clamoring over my head. That guy sticking his camera in your face at the cargo crawl or high-low line at Warrior Dash could've been me angling to preserve every bit of your passion, pain, and perseverance in photos.

You see, I'm an obstacle racer, too, and happily racing right alongside of you while getting the inspiration to write a book for you. Heck, it's a book *about you*. Enjoy what this book has in store for you. You may learn something, read one of your quotes, or see your muddy mug in one of our photos.

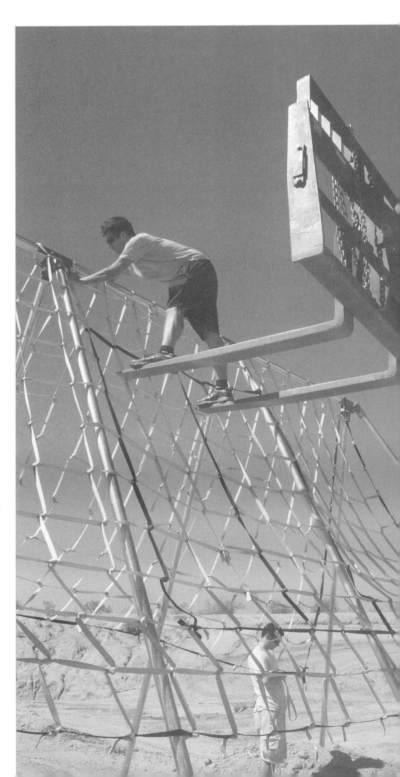

About This Book

Obstacle Race Training delves into the world of obstacle races and mud runs by providing in-depth reporting not only from adventures and challenges of all types but also from dedicated training facilities for athletes of all ages and levels. This is what you'll find in this book.

Part 1 describes the raucous, exciting, and challenging chaos of obstacle races and mud runs and covers the origins and history of these events. It also goes on to answer a very simple question: Why the hell would you do an obstacle race? The answers may surprise you! That big question is followed by a series of FAQs that we picked up during events and from race organizers and then wraps up with a complete Gear Guide to make sure you have the right stuff for race day.

For *Part 2*, I spent the better part of a year researching over 20 different races, interviewing the founders or race directors for each event, and even participating in as many events as my schedule would allow. Heck, on more than one occasion I actually worked with the event directors in setting up the obstacles pre-race! The behind-the-scenes look into the world of ob/mud adventures doesn't stop there—I dove into each of the events covered in this book to provide the inside scoop on each race's history, course methodology, and factors that make each one unique, exciting, and challenging.

Obstacle Race Training casts its net wide to capture all the categories in modern obstacle racing, including kids' events, women-only mud runs, timed events, challenges, themed events, zombies, and some events that are so ballistically extreme that only the best-of-the-best athletes even have the opportunity to be invited... and only an infinitesimally small percentage of them will survive to finish.

Now that you know what you're in for, you're ready for the training. In Part 3, I provide "Prepare to Dominate All Obstacles," the game plan to dominate any event and obstacle and strengthen your body by introducing you to the specific functional training you'll need to overcome any barriers between you and the finish line/beer garden. After providing step-by-step instruction, tips, and tricks to demolish any obstacle, I provide specific Strength, Dexterity, and Speed & Endurance exercises that are the foundation for the two-week Prep Program, the three-week Domination-Level Alpha Program, and the five-week CRUSH IT Program. I also give you the scoop on two very unique training facilities that prepare you for the challenges you may face during your obstacle race and mud run adventures. Once your body is ready, use the provided tips on how to prepare and test your gear about a week before your event and what to do on the morning of race day.

The *Appendix* features detailed descriptions and photos of all the stretches and additional exercises you'll need to perform the workouts.

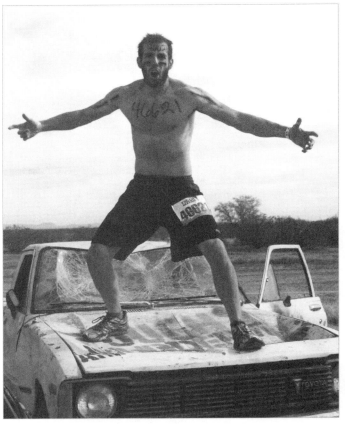

An enthusiastic participant showing a car who's boss at Tough Mudder.

What Is an Obstacle Race or Mud Run?

Obstacle races and mud runs come in many shapes, sizes, difficulties, and distances. On the most basic level, any event where impediments or challenges are placed on the course in the path of competitors is an obstacle race. According to Devon Anderson, founder of Cahoots Duo Challenge:

An obstacle race is equal parts mental toughness and physical endurance. These events require the primal desire to conquer the course and the physical dexterity to tackle each obstacle that we (happily) put in your way.

In a pure mud run, the primary obstacle is deep, thick, soupy, slimy mud that you need to navigate from start to finish—you won't find any walls or ropes at these events. These races are the human version of mud-bog tractor pulls, only you're providing all the horsepower. Equal parts running and mud slogging, these courses are notorious for saving the wettest, dirtiest element for the finish line, where you'll usually have to belly-crawl through a pit of mud to end the race.

Below is an overview of the landscape of these types of adventures and challenges. One thing that's for certain is they're all exciting and fun ways to spend a day racing with—or against—your friends.

When you're ready to have a dirty adventure of your own, check out www.mudrunguide.com, a comprehensive guide we've put together for you.

Puzzle-Solving/ Scavenger Races

Events that fall into the scavenger race category require some form of puzzle solving and orienteering. They also feature elements resembling a scavenger hunt played out on a grand scale (in some cases across an entire city). Occasionally these events can even take on the appearance of a pub crawl. When you show up for one of these types of events, expect to solve riddles, find clues, obtain pieces of puzzles, complete mental or physical challenges, and run (or hop on a bus or train), all the while trying to make it through all the checkpoints and to the finish line. (*Learn more about Scavenger Dash on page 51.*)

Racer vs. Obstacles

These events are based purely on defeating man-made or natural challenges and are all about speed, power, and finesse. You're judged solely by your time, so you need to figure out the fastest way over, under, around, and through each of the barriers that stand in your way in this all-out dash to the finish. Crawling over parked taxi cabs, climbing hundreds of stairs up a skyscraper, running up and down endless sand dunes, or scampering up, over, and down enormous cargo nets are just a taste of the types of obstacles you'll encounter. Course

DID YOU KNOW?

In 1995, the Eco-Challenge created by Mark Burnett was broadcast on MTV and ESPN as part of the X Games. The Eco-Challenge went on to be produced by and aired on the Discovery Channel from 1996 to 2000 and the USA Network until its demise in 2002.

lengths and designs differ widely. Men's Health Urbanathlon essentially covers a miniature city while other events are compact and/or parking-lot sized and have spectator-friendly courses. If you're looking for ice baths or mud puddles, check out "Hybrid Obstacle Races and Mud Runs" on page 13.

Racer vs. Course

In these types of events, the course fights back, with moving/changing obstacles and/or race staff who actively try to rattle you as you attempt to complete the course. Racers are pelted with water balloons, sprayed with hoses, and shot with paintball guns; they're forced to dodge swinging balls as they run through a gauntlet across balance beams suspended over water.

Events of this nature first grew into prominence on Japanese game shows where contestants are bounced, cajoled, and even pummeled while attempting to navigate safe passage through the course. Simpler, safer, and contestant-friendlier versions of these extreme obstacles soon found their way into the popular ABC show *Wipeout* or the much more physically demanding *American Ninja Warrior*. (*Learn more about ROC, the Ridiculous Obstacle Challenge on page 57, and Alpha Warrior on page 41.*)

Adventure Races

While some may call them the grandfather of obstacle races, adventure races are some of the most grueling endurance events in the world. They require map reading/orienteering and the use of various modes of transport, such as running, kayaking, mountain biking, rappelling, swimming, and horseback riding. They also involve tackling a host of obstacles, both natural and man-made. *(Learn more about adventure races in "The History behind Ob/Mud Events" on page 15.)*

Themed Events

Soldiers, knights, warriors, apocalyptic heroes, zombies, firefighters: Take your pick of the character you want to side with or even fight against when you enter a themed event. These races combine the challenge and excitement of an obstacle race with unique thematic elements plucked from movie sets or the demented minds of the event coordinators. Where else can you play the part of a damsel in distress, the hero, or even a sloppy bucket-of-flesh zombie? Each role has its own task. If you're lucky enough to find yourself in the ranks of the undead, your job is to track down and catch unwitting racers and eat their brains—well, rip off the flags from their belt as they try to squirm through the mudfest of a course on the way to the finish. *(Learn more about Run for Your Lives on page 56,* Hero Rush on page 55, and Obstacle Apocalypse on page 54.)

> "This sport has exploded in the last two years. It's expected to keep growing. It's no wonder why—it's sport and it's play all rolled into one. We don't just 'like' it, we 'need' it. We've created such an efficient world of order and rules and cubicles and structure. What we need sometimes is to run screaming in the other direction—in the direction of the mud."
> —Carrie Adams, founder, Rad Racing

Mud Runs

Hundreds of mud runs are held all over the world and that number is growing exponentially. From charity 5Ks to ultramarathon trail runs with river and swamp crossings to sprint-style events that feature little more than a parking lot's worth of running and a trough of mud before the finish line, there's a distance that'll fit anyone. Mud runs are not only growing rapidly in number of events, but with creative race directors on task, all events feature some twists on the basic formula (water + dirt = mud) and have taken on their own personality. *(Learn more about Del Mar Mud Run on page 44 and Mad Mud Run on page 45.)*

Hybrid Obstacle Races & Mud Runs

Once a cargo net or rope gets stretched over a mud pit, the line between a mud run and an obstacle race starts to blur and the event becomes a crossover sensation, a melting pot of awesomeness. There's no real name that sets these hybrids apart from their individual counterparts, hence the confusion for some racers showing up at events. The onus is on competitors to check out the website, read some reviews on Facebook or www.mudrunguide.com, and figure it out for themselves. Every race is different, so do your online homework first. No matter what, you're gonna have a hell of a great time.

These hybrids are the most prevalent events being held all over the world and draw their maniacal inspiration from all the events in the above list—some of the nastiest elements of adventure races mixed with huge man-made jungle gyms and natural impediments along with tons of goopy mud. Let's take a look at just a smattering of the types of challenges you'll face on these courses:

- Being submerged in an ice bath
- Hauling sand bags
- Lifting and dragging heavy rocks on a rope
- Traversing balance beams
- Climbing cargo nets
- Crawling under barbed wire
- Jumping over fire
- Braving electric shocks
- Jumping over, diving under, or crawling through barriers
- Scaling walls
- Scurrying up or swinging from ropes
- Throwing spears
- Leaping over or climbing hay bales (some may even be on fire)
- Running through or climbing over tires (lots and lots of tires)
- Scrambling over slippery walls covered in liquid soap
- Sloshing through streams, lakes, ponds, bogs, brooks, or even ditches or shipping containers filled with water
- Crawling through metric tons of mud
- Chopping wood
- Pulling yourself over wrecked cars

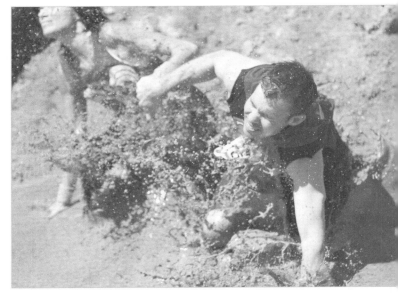

Teammates taking the leap into a Cahoots Duo Challenge mud pit.

By my count, that's about 25 great reasons to start looking to sign up for a hybrid obstacle race and mud run right now! Starting on page 32 in "Obstacle Races, Mud Runs, and Extreme Challenges," I list 25 more exciting and difficult obstacles and highlight over a dozen of the biggest, baddest, and most exhilarating events in the world. *(Learn more about Spartan Race on page 34, Tough Mudder on page 39, Savage Race on page 37, Warrior Dash on page 36, and Rugged Maniac on page 38.)*

"A quality obstacle course should never let you get into a comfort zone; it should keep you on your toes and continually present new challenges, both mental and physical. If you can hold yourself together during an obstacle race, you can hold yourself together in life."
—Michael Sandercock, founder, Obstacleracers.com

The History behind Ob/Mud Events

While obstacle racing and mud runs are currently the hottest and fastest-growing sports around the globe, they're in no way considered new additions to the world of athletics and training. Since the beginning of wars and conflicts, soldiers have needed combat training, which means new recruits have been climbing ropes and cargo nets, scaling walls, slogging through mud and water, and trekking over arduous terrain since the dawn of man. Prior to humans, velociraptors dominated the Jurassic Games,[1] and were relatively unstoppable when it came to agility and speed...but that's a whole different topic for another time.

---

1 T-Rex hated cargo nets, look it up.

Military Boot Camp

The earliest evidence of organized military training can be traced back to the Persians, who developed extensive training regimens for warriors to hone their strength, skills, and wits in order to survive combat and emerge victorious from battle. Recruits would be trained and tested for up to ten years before being allowed to enlist in the Persian Army. The Greeks were famous for developing their recruits' physical fitness and skill, and the development of Roman Army training yielded a soldier that was equally smart and strong in order to grasp the intricacies of warfare and tactics.

Over the last couple of centuries, military preparedness has advanced significantly due to the focus on effective training methods to the point where current recruits in developed countries are benefitted by huge financial, logistical, and time investments into modern boot camps. The term "boot camp" was coined prior to World War I by Sergeant Major Matthew A. Gaskgar[2] of the 121st Airborne in reference to Camp Booth in Lewiston Maine, where as a youth he would spend his summers sitting in the sun by the lake weaving baskets...of course that's a lie! Boot camp, basic training, recruit training—whatever term you choose refers to the hundreds of hours that "grunts" spend tromping through all types of conditions to prepare for the rigors of battle, all the while counting on their boots as their prized possessions to keep their feet protected. Quite simply put: Soldiers who can't walk can't fight.

Military training around the globe has come a long way from the decade-long Persian Army version and is on average eight to sixteen weeks in duration, focusing on discipline, leadership,

intense physical fitness, weapons training, hand-to-hand combat, first aid, survival training, and teamwork. Soldiers must be able to handle themselves in any situation, and there's nothing better than "Hell Week" to get them ready for that challenge.

The first week of boot camp is commonly referred to as "Hell Week" in the U.S. armed forces. Each recruit is pushed to the edge of his or her mental and physical limits with strenuous activities such as extremely long marches through difficult terrain with little or no sleep for days on end. In elite camps like Navy SEAL training, trainees perform 132 hours straight of physical activity with no sleep; it's no surprise that nearly 80 percent of recruits drop out in the first phase of training. Only the truly elite students who can survive and pass through this grueling training emerge as Special Forces soldiers.

It's from these elite military training camps that several obstacle races and mud runs have been forged. One well-known example is the Camp Pendleton World Famous Mud Run.

Located on 125,000 acres in San Diego, California, and bordering the crisp, clear waters of the Pacific Ocean and some of Southern California's signature pristine beaches, Camp Pendleton is the site of one of America's toughest challenges: qualifying to become a

---

It should be no surprise at all that some soldiers relish the torture, hardship, and abuse that they endured while in basic training and crave the hard-fought victory of surviving and thriving in such a harsh environment. The influence of military service and even Special Forces training is visible in the development of obstacle races and mud runs all over the world; numerous race directors, founders, and contributors to obstacle races and mud runs large and small have a strong military background.

---

2 Matt A Gaskgar = Madagascar. Totally fictional character

Heads were burning in the unique conditions of sunny warmth and ice-covered water. Thus you experienced the sensation of severe instant headache as your hot blood rushed to your head and exploded as you ducked into the underwater pool and tunnel. One brave contestant said he now knew what hell was like and would be a good boy for the rest of his life!

—Tough Guy Jelly Leg News, 1997

U.S. Marine. The amazing scenery belies the torturous challenges awaiting all new recruits when they set foot on these hallowed grounds, where thousands of Marines have been forged over the last 70 years. Created to challenge cadets, Camp Pendleton's gates are opened a few times a year for civilians to test their mettle on the demanding course as well as other challenges, ranging from 5Ks to half marathons. At the end of the day, the dog tag–shaped finisher's medals on their chest will not be the same as those brave soldiers who earned their stripes as Marines, but the feeling of victory and accomplishment is second to none—at least, once you wipe the mud from your face and get a celebratory beer in your hand.

TOUGH GUY—FROM THE MIND OF A MOUSE

Over the last 25 years, one obstacle race has pioneered many of the obstacles, barriers, and dastardly pitfalls that are re-created in obstacle races and mud runs all over the globe. Most events will give a tip of their cap to Billy Wilson (a.k.a. Mr. Mouse) as being the godfather of the sport and the impetus for creating their own challenging courses in an attempt to share some of the Tough Guy spirit and glory all over the world. Tough Guy was the origin of obstacle racing, the first organized event of its type, where civilians could challenge themselves on military-style courses. It has earned a special

place in history—and in this book—as being a big reason why this sport even exists today.

Tough Guy events are as brutal as its race director is colorful. The events held in summer are extremely difficult, and the winter version is downright ridiculous when the temperatures plummet and the water crossings turn to ice. In 2010, over 600 competitors were treated for hypothermia and thousands others finished the event with bumps, bruises, and scratches to go along with their immense sense of accomplishment on having finished a true original and what some call the toughest challenge in the world of adventure sports.

Devon Anderson, founder of Cahoots Duo Challenge, relates his first encounter with Tough Guy: "A mysterious hush falls over the crowd; competitors abruptly end their conversations, forget about their pre-race jitters, and look around to see what is going on. Walking up the crest of 'Trample Hill' to the right of the throngs of would-be racers is a shadowy figure seemly plucked from a WWII battlefield, an elderly yet sturdy gentleman who has donned a kilt and military uniform with a huge white bushy mustache flapping against a wrinkled and determined face illuminated as the rising sun burns off the morning fog. Mumbled tales are whispered from racer to racer as to whether he is mortal or merely an apparition that has been haunting these grounds for eons. 'I heard he's over a hundred years old' mixes with 'He runs this course every morning for the fun of it' as the awestruck competitors blink and rub their eyes in an attempt to get a clearer view of this mesmerizing superhero perched above them, surveying each one of the huddled hopefuls below. As slowly and deliberately as a general might, he raises his arm in an apparent move to wave his soldiers off to battle. He pauses briefly, and then brings his arm down like a hammer as he has done for 25 years. A loud 'boom' from the cannon and the gates open; the Tough Guy battle has begun and multiple hours of torture are now underway before the strongest and bravest of competitors can claim their place as a Tough Guy finisher."

(Learn more about Tough Guy on page 64 and Cahoots Duo Challenge on page 50.

Adventure Racing

Created by TV producer Mark Burnett (*Survivor, The Apprentice*), Eco-Challenge was the first worldwide adventure race and is considered by many to have put the sport on the global radar. From 1995 to 2002, the format was refined and tweaked in an attempt to make events more difficult, exciting, and TV-friendly, in the process defining adventure racing as an entirely self-encompassing sport featuring a mix of multiple disciplines. The term "adventure race" was coined by journalist Martin Dugard when he described the discipline required by athletes to conquer the challenges in events such as Eco-Challenge.

Probably the most well-known adventure race was Primal Quest, held six times between 2002 and 2009. PQ courses traversed 400-plus miles and lasted for up to 10 days, during which co-ed teams of four battled the course, the elements, and other competitors without the aid of support crews or navigational assistance. Each of the six PQ courses featured incredibly picturesque yet difficult terrain, with mountain ascents and descents in sub-freezing climates and treks through hundreds of miles of barren wasteland where the mercury topped out over 110 degrees. Participant and crew safety as well as the immense costs of conducting an adventure race on such a grand scale was responsible for the limited number of events held, as was the unfortunate death of an extremely experienced adventure racer, Nigel Aylott, in 2004. PQ holds the distinction as being the first expedition adventure race to be broadcast on television, with highlights shown on CBS in 2004 and 2005, and ESPN and ABC providing coverage in 2006.

Hundreds of smaller adventure race events, with distances ranging from 10 to 60 miles and durations between 4 to 24 hours, are held all over the world every year to challenge the small yet dedicated following of adventure-racing athletes. The United States Adventure Racing Association (USARA) currently sanctions events throughout the U.S. and features a point system for ranking teams seeking to qualify for the 24-hour national championship.

Why the Hell Would You Do an Obstacle Race?

Why? *Because you can.* Obstacle races and mud runs have something for everyone and are wide open to anyone willing to sign up, show up, and never give up. It's a primal desire inside of all of us to go outside and play in the mud, get dirty, and have a blast with our friends. The barriers to entry are very low or relatively nonexistent at many obstacle races and mud runs, and so much easier to compete in when compared to nearly every other organized event you can sign up for.

Obstacle races and mud runs are the ultimate weekend-warrior event. People of all ages, sizes, backgrounds, and athletic ability come together to play in the mud, have fun, and push their limits. Most aren't showing up to win—the simple glory of competing is a triumph in and of itself.

ADVENTURE RACES	TRIATHLONS	MARATHONS	BIKE RACING	ORGANIZED SPORTS
Require orienteering, mountain biking, mountain climbing and rappelling, running, endurance, skill, and a tremendous amount of tolerance for blisters	Require swimming, biking, running, a wetsuit, skin-tight clothing, goofy swim goggles, bike helmets, and shaved legs	Require running 26.2 miles	Requires costly two-wheeled contraptions, shaved legs, and tight outfits (see also: Triathlons)	Require equipment, field, goals, and sport-specific skill. Can you hit a curve ball at 85 mph? What about returning a tennis serve at 120 mph? Dunk a basketball?

Find an event in your area, talk some of your buddies into signing up, pull together an outfit that you don't mind ruining, and go get muddy! During the development of this book there were literally thousands of different viewpoints that went into the descriptions of these events, but the only way you'll have any clue how fun and exciting they can be is if you sign up, show up, and get dirty!

Before You Sign Up

The very first thing you should do before signing up for any event is to get your lazy ass checked out by a doctor. Seriously, no one wants to see you get carted off the course by EMTs because you weren't healthy enough to sign up in the first place. Once you get the green light from your doc, spend some time checking out the event's website. Review the distance and conditions to get a good idea of what you're in for when you show up on race day—if you still have the guts to sign up.

Pay special attention to the rules. It's your responsibility to know what's expected of you on the course. No, you can't fight back against the zombies chasing you, and impersonating Chuck Norris with a spinning back kick to a gladiator

is not allowed. Some events will give you recommendations on clothing or gear to wear. If they don't offer that info, you can check out the "Gear Guide" on page 26.

Getting your body and mind ready to compete is the most important element of pre-race preparation. Some events are a fun excuse to get mud in a few hard-to-reach crevices of your body and afterward have a beer with your friends, while others are extremely challenging endeavors that'll test your physical and mental fortitude. If you're signing up for the latter, it's important to prepare for some of the rigors you'll encounter on race day by running, exercising, and even taking an ice-cold shower or two. In Part 3 (page 68), you'll find "Training to Crush the World's Most Bad-Ass Courses" program, where we'll prepare you to dominate all obstacles. You'll find dozens of tips, tricks, techniques, and real-life exercises you can use to get ready to tackle some of the most common obstacles you'll find on race day. In "Mental Preparation: What the Hell Are You Thinking?" (page 109) we'll cover the mental aspect of signing up, showing up, and toeing the line to take on these amazing challenges.

Frequently Asked Questions

Q: Can I really do a mud run?

A: Um, yeah. In the immortal words of Patches O'Houlihan, "If you can dodge a wrench, you can dodge a ball." Let's expand on that sound logic a bit: "If you can run, walk, or even crawl from the start to the finish, you can complete a mud run."

Basically, if you can walk approximately 3 miles in muddy clothes, you can complete your first mud run. It may not be pretty, but that first taste of victory is usually all it takes to turn your average couch potato into an addicted mud runner. That's why this sport is ballooning to epic proportions, with new events being added worldwide nearly every day.

Q: What type of training do I need to complete an obstacle race or mud run?

A: Athletes don't necessarily "need" training… wait—don't put the book down! YES, YOU NEED TRAINING! (Whew, that was close!) While everyone meeting the minimum age requirements is welcome at most events, you should have a baseline level of fitness that'll allow you to participate safely and not be an undue burden on those around you or block their path. The code of honor at nearly every event is to help those around you at each obstacle to your best ability prior to moving on, and that's extremely difficult to do with individuals who lack the strength, know-how, or fortitude to help themselves. Starting on page 69 we cover obstacle-specific techniques, tips, exercises, and specific training programs to develop your strength, dexterity, speed, and endurance in order to crush the world's most bad-ass courses.

Q: How do I prepare for the obstacles I'm going to face?

A: Well, how many times have you climbed a cargo net? Scaled an eight-foot wall? Jumped over flaming hay bales? Until you've completed your first obstacle race or hell week in military training, the answer is most likely zero. On race day, you're only going to have a few seconds to decide how to tackle an obstacle that you most likely have never seen before. Sometimes that ends with either your body or ego in a bumped and bruised mess crumbled at the base of a barrier. On page 69 in "Prepare to Dominate All Obstacles," we cover different barriers, challenges, and obstacles and show you step by step how to prepare your mind and body to be able to crush each of them.

Q: What's the best way to get into competing in obstacle races?

A: Volunteer at an event! You'll learn more about the passion and excitement coursing through every competitor's veins and get some useful behind-the-scenes knowledge that you can use when you tackle the course yourself. Yeah, you'll be out there for hours at a time and maybe get grimy, sweaty, sunburned, or even a little frostbitten, but you're right there and part of the action. If that isn't enough motivation to get you to volunteer, consider this: Most events give steep discounts or even free entry to volunteers! Check with your race for their policy before you sign up. Oh, yeah…you also may get a chance to be a zombie.

Q: What should I wear?

A: While nudity is not permitted at any of the major events, men in thongs seem to converge by the dozens to participate in mud runs. This attire is not only permitted, it's encouraged in the form of prizes for costumes: the best, the worst, the skimpiest, etc. A word of warning about costumes—what you wear to the start line will be in tatters by the finish. If you start out with a tutu and angel wings, you'll be dragging those sodden wings through every obstacle and mud pit and dealing with the chafing from your decorative tutu every step of the way.

Almost all costumes fall way short on protecting the areas of your body that take the most abuse during an event: your elbows, knees, hands, forearms, shins, and feet. Covering yourself head to toe with protective garments may be a little too excessive, so your best bet is choosing an outfit somewhere in

"Jumping, crawling, and climbing are all things we're naturally born to do....We're wired to do them, but we don't anymore; we just type."

—Joe DeSena, founder, Death Race

between. Check out the "Gear Guide" on page 26.

Q: How "in shape" should I be?

A: Aside from extreme invite-only events, all obstacle races and mud runs are suitable for most athletes of any size, shape, and ability. Of course, you're required to sign a waiver that states you're healthy enough to participate and have been checked out and cleared by a medical professional before attempting any event. At any race you'll see a diverse cross-section of fitness levels and body types. If you have the willpower to finish, there's a spot for you at nearly every starting line.

Q: What is the easiest type of event?

A: "Easy" is a relative term, but the majority of mud runs are less demanding than obstacle races and feature far fewer (if any) barriers other than mud, terrain, and more mud. That being said, every single course will feature terrain or challenges that are unique and will test your mental and physical toughness...or at least your ability to laugh at yourself!

Q: So what's the toughest course out there?

A: All of them. Every single course is a challenge and, based on your particular strengths, even the shortest course may be particularly demanding based on the obstacles laid out by the race organizers. Toughness is also relative to the individual racer: If you

struggle with running, the longer distances may prove to be extremely daunting; if you have weak upper-body strength, events that require a lot of hanging, swinging, or rope climbing could be your undoing. A well-rounded course will have plenty of barriers standing between you and an "easy" run. Every single course is so dramatically different that there's no effective way that I know of to rank them against each other in terms of toughness. With the sport of obstacle racing constantly evolving, new obstacles are created daily and added to the repertoire of talented (and somewhat masochistic) race directors. Joe DeSena of Spartan Race (which features courses in a multitude of lengths) confided in me that the shorter the overall course distance is, the harder they make each of the obstacles!

If you're looking for an answer about which events are the most difficult, that's a little easier to define. Any event that requires you to qualify to compete is generally too difficult for the average weekend warrior. These "invite-only" events include (but are not limited to):

Death Race—A 24- to 70-hour endurance event composed of mud runs, obstacle racing, trail racing, physical challenges, and mental challenges where 90% of the entrants will not finish. Based on "life lesson" themes, each year the event is diabolically designed to break each competitor mentally and physically.

World's Toughest Mudder—An extreme mud run open to the top finishers of Tough Mudder events all over the world. To win, an athlete has to complete the most loops of the Tough Mudder course in 24 hours. After that, all other entrants are given four additional hours to complete an equal number of laps to be considered finishers.

Spartan Ultra Beast—The world's first marathon-distance obstacle race, this 26.2-mile course is two loops of the Spartan Beast course and dubbed the most difficult Spartan Race course ever.

Tough Guy UK—Often imitated, never duplicated, this event is held twice a year on the second Sunday in July and last Sunday in January. The summer "Nettle Warrior" version is nearly double the length of the winter version, yet only completing the latter is considered a true Tough Guy accomplishment.

Check out the extreme challenges on page 62 for more info on these events.

Q: Are there events for first-timers?

A: Yes—every event is for first-timers! The enormous growth and popularity of the sport guarantees that there'll be hundreds—if not thousands—of first-timers at most events. Even if you've raced another mud run or obstacle race before, each course features different obstacles, distances, and terrain. So every time everyone shows up for an event, it's arguably everyone's "first time."

As a first-timer, the best advice is to pick a start time that'll give you the opportunity to scout the course—if you're allowed—and surround yourself with other racers who are the same general ability as you. When lining up for your start, move toward the back of the pack so you can observe others tackling each obstacle. Build your confidence as you conquer the race elements and then you can pick up the pace. Sprinting out of the starting gate isn't the best option—take your time and absorb the lessons from the competitors in front of you. Let them wade into the mud first and you can pick your

path based on immediate feedback from their results.

Q: Can I compete with a team?

A: Absolutely. Showing up on race day with a team is not only encouraged by race staff, it's a fantastic way to show that handsome guy from accounting that everyone's equal when they're adorned in muck. Seriously, participating with a team is extremely beneficial for first-timers, as you have a built-in cheering squad and support staff on every obstacle. Make sure you do your part for the group and help out as much as you get helped—or more. The best part about being in a team may be the matching costumes or T-shirts, but team registrations may also get a discount, so check your race's website.

Q: If I can't get over an obstacle, what can I do?

A: Let's break it down into steps:

Step 1: Assess the obstacle before engaging; figure out its weaknesses and the elements of the barrier you can use. Are there stanchions or supports you could use to boost yourself up? Is one side easier to climb/descend/crawl through than the other?

Step 2: Watch other competitors and their success or failures and take notes. It also won't hurt your karma if you help them out, and you just might get the same treatment from other competitors.

Step 3: Engage the obstacle and commit to conquering it; this means use your momentum, strength, and every bit of your mental fortitude to crush that obstacle. Every wall that you half-heartedly attempted to climb is a waste of your energy as you'll have to try again after you fail.

Step 4: Didn't tackle it? Follow steps 1–3 again. There may be a trick that you need to figure out in order to pass.

Step 5: If you've made it to this step and you're still not past the obstacle, you probably didn't take the hint in step #2 about getting good karma by helping someone else—so go do it! Follow the Dirty Rule: *Do unto other mud runners as you would have them do unto you.* If you need to ask for help, don't be shy. Who knows, that person may need your help on the next obstacle, and maybe they'll even write you into their will in the event of a real zombie apocalypse. You'll never know unless you ask.

Step 6: Hi...you're still here? OK, this would be a good time to chalk this obstacle up to "I'll get it next time" and bypass it carefully. If this is a timed event, you may have to pay a penalty like doing burpees or push-ups, but at least you're getting a good (forced) workout. As you pass, take one last look at that menacing barrier between you and immortality and vow to yourself that you'll one day emerge victorious. Now, wipe that mud off your face and soldier on to the next obstacle!

Q: The event I signed up for has a "wave start." What does that mean?

A: In events with large numbers of competitors, the race organizers will break down the racers into groups with more manageable numbers and stagger their start time. This allows for a more enjoyable experience for participants and less overcrowding or waiting at obstacles. An interval of 10 to 15 minutes is common between groups, depending on the size of the course, number of obstacles, and race-day conditions.

Some of the largest events have adopted the practice of assigning exact start times spaced throughout the day. Not only does this cut down on course congestion but it also allows racers to relax, spectate, and prepare for the event without worrying about what wave they'll be in. As a practice, the fastest or "elite" competitors will get the earliest start times and be challenged by a course that hasn't been trodden upon by thousands of racers.

Q: Are all events timed?

A: No, not all events are timed. Some are classified as "races" and others as "challenges." One isn't better than the other, just different. Courses that are timed are usually geared a little differently than untimed ones. Pick the ones that are right for you.

Q: Is obstacle racing just a fad?

A: Let's ask Carrie Adams: "I don't believe obstacle racing is a fad. In fact, I hope it's a sign of things to come and that we're rediscovering what it feels like being our most physical selves. Abandon the desk, the couch, and even the pavement. Go off road and find out what's beyond the things that you can easily see."

Q: Will zombies really chase me through the woods trying to eat my brains?

A: Yes, they'll chase you and, no, your brains are safe. They're merely trying to rip the flags dangling from your race belt.

Q: Do you have to be totally nuts to enjoy mud runs and obstacle races?

A: No, but it surely helps.

Gear Guide

If there's mud or water on the course, cotton is the enemy. Whether it's in your shirt, shoes, shorts socks, or underwear, cotton will absorb the wetness (and muck) and you'll be left with that oh-so-satisfying feeling of wearing an adult diaper. Take a tip from triathletes when you're getting dressed: Synthetic fibers in body-hugging designs make the fastest and most efficient outfits. By that same token, the Borat-style man-sling costume is not necessarily that bad of an idea...but I digress.

Loose-fitting clothes can get snagged on obstacles, grabbed accidentally (or not) by other racers, and even obscure your view. Chafing, blisters, and a couple hours of discomfort could be unwelcome additions to your race if you choose the wrong gear or a wickedly uncomfortable costume.

Follow the KISS principle—keep it simple, stupid. A minimal outfit with less things to worry about allows you to focus on the course. If you're wearing a costume, it's all up to you; don't let the rules of good taste stand in the way of your tutu.

Shoes: Your shoes should be well-fitting athletic models in order to prevent blisters. Aggressive tread (NOT cleats, they're not allowed in any race I've interviewed, so leave them at home) with thin, slick material on the upper so they don't hold excess water or mud are preferable. Keeping your feet as light as possible, with minimal mud coming along for a free ride, is beneficial, as you'll be lifting your paws up about 6,000 times on a 5K course and you'll begin to feel every single extra ounce.

There are even some quasi-obstacle-race-specific models on the market from Innov-8, Columbia, New Balance, and Merrell that feature all the grip you need along with an upper and/or sole that drains water quickly. Check out the Gear Guide on www.mudrunguide.com/gear for our top picks and reviews.

Want to test your shoes before you hit the race course? In "Getting Ready to Race" (page 129), we give advice on how to test your shoe and sock choice out to prevent blisters on the big day.

Socks: No matter how much effort and cash you put into getting your shirt, shorts, and shoes all set, all that's for moot if you don't follow this simple advice: *Do not wear cotton socks if there's even a drop of water on the course.* The extra moisture held by cotton coupled with running or walking will most likely leave you with blisters. Wet cotton also loses its shape easily, so your socks will rub in places you'd never expect as well as slip out of place on your ankle and let rocks, dirt, and debris in.

Looking to find some good events? You only need to go to one place to see all the crazy events you're going to talk your co-worker's ears off about for the next year. We developed www.mudrunguide.com so you can search for, review, and sign up for obstacle races and mud runs all over the world. Yeah, you're welcome.

Pick up a pair of man-made-fiber socks that fit snugly above your ankles; they'll drain faster coupled with good shoes and keep the junk out of the inside of your socks.

Gaiters: Endurance trail runners swear by them, and they can be extremely helpful to keep dirt, rocks, and debris out of your shoes when running over rough terrain, but they're a personal decision as they can be expensive and a bit of a pain to get fitted properly. A good, albeit ugly, solution is to buy an extra-large pair of man-made-fiber tube socks, cut the toes off, and slip them over the heel of your shoe and up your ankle. Duct tape the bottom to your heel and around the laces of your shoes; experiment with fit and test them out ahead of time.

Shirts: Yeah, it's very cool to get matching silk-screened T-shirts for your entire team. The only problem is that most of the time the cheapest and most readily available customized shirts are cotton, and we've already covered why those suck in the mud. Now, we're not advocating writing "Mud Puppy Marauders" on the front and back of eight different $59 Under Armour tech jerseys, but a tight-fitting, man-made-fabric top would probably be the best course of action. The other is to go shirtless (dudes) or sports-bra/jogging top (ladies).

Shorts/Pants: "Do as I say, not as I do" Part I: Make sure your pants can stay up on their own! I made the mistake of wearing loose-fitting cargo shorts at a Spartan Race and ended up in my spandex underwear by mile number three. Cargo shorts or pants with pockets are a relatively bad idea—anything that can fill with mud *will* fill with mud. Basketball shorts, even if they're made of synthetic materials, are usually a bad idea as they can be heavy, long, and have pockets. Medium-length running shorts are a good choice; they dry quickly, are light, and most likely won't be down around your ankles when you're scooting under barbed wire. If the weather's cooler, warm-up nylon pants are great, as their slick surface will give you a little advantage when you're on your belly writhing in the mud. They'll also keep your knees from turning into hamburger from contact with the dirt.

Gloves: Usually the most hotly debated question the morning of an event or on blogs and Facebook is whether you should wear gloves or not. The answer is simple: Wear them for obstacles that are nasty on your hands (pulling/climbing ropes, carrying rough objects like cinder blocks, logs, or anything that requires a good grip) and take them off and shove them in a pocket or down the back of your pants when you don't need them. Make sure the gloves fit your hands very well and have plenty of grip; avoid leather or anything that can get slick or hold water. Fingerless workout gloves are commonly found on the course because they get wet and slick and actually make it harder to grip smooth surfaces like monkey bars. Gardening gloves that look like someone dipped a basic pair of fabric gloves into molten rubber work really well and are relatively cheap; check out our gear guide on www.mudrunguide.com/gear for reviews and suggestions.

Knee/Elbow Pads or Neoprene Sleeves: Protecting your knees, elbows, and hands is a very good idea. Most events will have at least a half-dozen obstacles specifically designed to have you crawling on those tender areas and it's a good idea to protect them if you'd like to finish the race with all your skin. Leave the rollerblade hardshell pads at home and opt for thin knee or elbow pads or simple neoprene sleeves. I prefer the latter to cover my knees and elbows as they provide enough cushioning when I run into an obstacle and enough protection to crawl through mud, tubes, and anything else the course has to throw at me while still allowing me the full range of motion to run.

Costumes: An entire book could be written just on the dos and don'ts of costumes and the perilous outcomes of really bad comical attire decisions. Yes, costumes are funny and proclaim your independent (usually cross-dressing) spirit, and there's a one-in-five thousand or so chance that you'll win a $50 gift card to Chili's for dressing like Dorothy with Toto in a basket stapled onto your back.

"Do as I say, not as I do" Part II: Yes, I've been seen with fairy wings and a tutu at Mad Mud Run. No, I didn't win a prize (dammit!) and the chafing from the wings and halo-in-the-eyes wasn't worth it. Yeah, I included the photo—that's me on the left side of the photo.

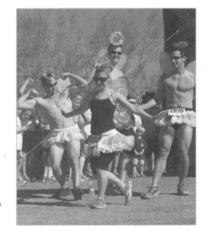

Whatever you wear to the race is what you'll be dealing with the entire event, whether that's running, crawling, climbing, bending, or even sometimes swimming. If you flaunt the KISS rules, then you've got to deal with it. Anything that can fall apart will fall apart. Anything that can chafe will chafe. Anything that looks cool at the beginning of the race will look like a mess at the end of the race.

Ear/Nose Plugs and Goggles:
Anywhere that can hold mud will eventually get packed with it. Emptying mud out of your pockets or from inside your shoes is much easier than cleaning it out of your ENT orifices, your ears especially. Each event I do that features mud results in dirty Q-tips for a week after showers and can easily be avoided by packing your ears with a quality disposable pair of ear plugs. Just say no to nose plugs—I've never seen them on the course and it's pretty easy to use the "snot rocket" technique to clear a mud-packed nostril quickly.

"Here's mud in your eye," my ass. There's nothing particularly enjoyable about getting your eyes full of mud. I can personally attest to how much I hated life immediately after finishing Warrior Dash AZ in 2012 when I gave everything I had in the mud pit to catch up to the guy who was just seconds in front of me in first place and filled every square millimeter of my orbital cavity with fresh, thick, Florence, Arizona, mud. Not only did I finish second in my heat, but my eyes burned for the 100-mile ride home and even a few hours afterward. Yes, I'd do it all over again and, no, I still wouldn't wear goggles, but that's just me. If you have sensitive eyes or contact lenses or don't want to show up to the office on Monday like you spent the weekend with Jeff Spicoli (see *Fast Times at Ridgemont High*), then popping a pair of swimmer's goggles on right before the mud pit is an option. But don't wear them the whole race—you'll just look silly.

Stuff: "Attention, racers, if you find an iPhone in a pink case out on the course, there's a $100 reward for the person who turns it in

> "Wearing a race's shirt while you're running that race is like wearing a band's shirt to that band's concert. We know you like the race—you're running it. Save the shirt for after you cross the finish line and toss your muddy clothes."
> —Michael Sandercock, founder, Obstacleracers.com

to an official on the course. Please do not put it in your pocket and run through the water obstacles. Thank you." —Announcer at Spartan Race AZ 2012.

If you don't want to lose it, then don't bring it on the course. Your cellphone and wallet belong in the car after registration is done. Your earrings, necklaces, and anything that's worth more than $5 that's clipped, strapped, draped, or hung around your body will fall off and be gone forever—it's as simple as that. There are some awesome and honest race volunteers out there who may give you your smartphone back, but why should they have to carry your stuff around? Be responsible and leave anything that isn't required for the race in your locked car or checked gear bag (although you should never leave valuables in your gear bag, just a change of clothes and maybe a backup set of car keys).

Waterproof, head-mounted video recorders are OK-ish, but be prepared to edit out all the shots looking up the leg of someone's shorts during an obstacle and getting an eyeful of something that you had no intention of seeing the first time, never mind playing it back on tape. My personal opinion is to go out and run the race and leave the videography to the people who do it for a living, such as Jon, who happens to film great race footage for us at www.mudrunguide.com.

PART 2: EVENTS

Obstacle Races, Mud Runs, & Extreme Challenges

Here's my favorite definition of obstacle races and mud runs from Carrie Adams of Rad Racing: "Obstacle racing mixes road racing, trail running, and cross-country running with a variety of obstacles throughout the course to test endurance, strength, speed, and dexterity...There's something so empowering about the not knowing what's next in a race like this, about just surviving the next step, overcoming the next obstacle. Your breath, your lungs, your heart beating in your chest...when you're on the course, it's not just living—it's being *alive*. There's a huge difference, and you'll only realize it if you're willing to push yourself to your limits."

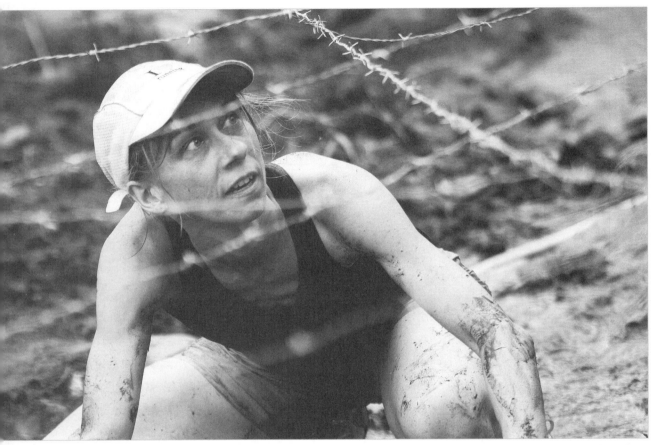

Barbed wire is the least of your worries at the Death Race.

Running from zombies, swinging across monkey bars, jumping rope, diving into water from high platforms, cruising down zip lines, crossing parallel bars, avoiding gladiators smacking you with pugil sticks, being shot at with paintball guns, getting pelted with water balloons or sprayed with hoses, bombing down slip and slides or muddy hills into swamps, crawling through muddy tubes, scampering over horizontal climbing walls, balance beams, evading sharks (just checking to see if you were paying attention), carrying sandbags, climbing rope ladders, crawling up muddy slopes, running through mazes and dirty, dusty, and hilly trails, swimming through icy water, rope-climbing over walls—these are just a few combinations of jumping, crawling, dodging, and sprinting that await you on some of the most creative courses and terrain imaginable.

Back on page 14, we posted about 25 challenging, dirty, and exciting obstacles that are waiting for you on race day at some—or all—of the mud runs and obstacle races listed on the following pages. Here's an additional bunch to whet your appetite a bit more.

Obstacle Races: Are You Tough Enough?

Varying in length from 5 kilometers to 12 miles, the obstacle races in this section are much more demanding than any "fun mud run." Dozens of dastardly obstacles wait around every corner of the course to stall, challenge, and frustrate even the fittest and most adept racer. Natural barriers of fire, ice, and mud, along with nasty terrain, are augmented by man-made structures designed to test the mettle of every single athlete who dreams of finish-line glory. Make no mistake about it, these are some of the most bad-ass courses on the planet.

Spartan Race

Multi-distance obstacle race, worldwide locations

Launched: 2010

Events: 29 in 2012, 36+ in 2013

Kids' Events: Junior Spartan, ages 4–9; Varsity Spartan, ages 10–13

Course Distances: Sprint 5K, Super 10K, Beast 20K

Obstacles: More than a dozen; course layout is not revealed prior to race—"it's like life, you don't know what's coming next"

Terrain: Varies by location depending on topography; course will use any and all natural obstacles and elements to make a demanding and interesting course

Signature Obstacle: Gladiator Arena: before the finish line, athletes must pass through "gladiators" who try to knock down runners using their pugil sticks

Hardest Obstacle: Spear throw—if (or when) you miss the target, 30 burpees are waiting for you. There are many more physically demanding obstacles on the course, but the failure rate at the spear throw is extremely high

Penalties: Failing or skipping any obstacle results in a penalty of 30 burpees

Gear: Wear athletic gear that'll allow movement in any direction as you'll be climbing over and scurrying under obstacles, lifting and pulling heavy objects, running trails through water and mud, and jumping over fire. Gloves may help with some rope-based obstacles; well-fitting athletic shoes should help minimize blisters

Founded by an Englishman, a Canadian, and some of the most prolifically demanding race

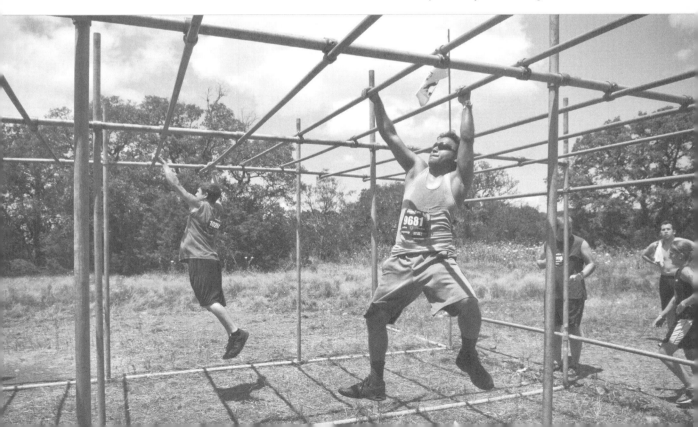

directors America has ever seen, Spartan Race is at once a brutally demanding challenge as well as a fun, exciting event with finishers of all ages and fitness levels. The race started by a chance encounter in the little town of Pittsfield, Vermont, when the aforementioned Canadian (Selica) and Englishman (Richard) emerged from hiking the Appalachian Trail for about three months and met Joe DeSena, who dared them to compete in Death Race—one of the most demanding endurance events on the planet—the following day. Richard, an ex–Royal Marine and ultra athlete, convinced Selica to give it a go and, after a few hours of scrounging gear from some charitable locals, they took their place at the starting line. Against some of the toughest competition from nearly 200 ultra athletes, Selica was the last woman standing after 10 hours before she had to drop out, having succumbed to hypothermia. Richard did slightly better—he won the damn thing. (Actually, he was a co-winner, but that's not integral to this story. Learn more about Death Race on page 66). Undeterred from her unsuccessful first attempt, Selica returned to Death Race the following year and finished in third place.

Says Selica, "We wanted everyone to feel what we're feeling at that moment, the incredible sense of accomplishment, the rush of emotions, the amazing excitement and adrenaline rush from being challenged...we needed to bring this to everyone, even if it's only for a day."

Richard and Selica teamed up with Death Race nutjobs Joe and Andy Weinberg and decided to bring this concept to the masses: the ultimate human sport that brought people back to their roots. Climbing, crawling, jumping, swimming, combat, defying fire and naturally

> "Obstacle racing is a metaphor for life...when you are born, no one gives you a map to your life journey, nor what obstacles you will overcome. It is those who adapt, who are strong both mentally and physically, and of course who have a sense of humor, who survive."
> —Selica Sevigny, co-founder, Spartan Race

occurring obstacles—adventures and hardships that humans have dealt with for eons. Ultra athletes and exceptional race directors such as Andy Weinberg, Noel Hannah, Mike Morris, and Brian Duncanson contributed to the evolution of the race and the idea of the ultimate obstacle race series was born.

According to the directors, "Spartan Race's mission from the beginning was to have various levels so people could work their way up by building their strength and confidence. We created a new sport with specific distances: Sprint 5K, Super 10K, Beast 20K. We created a world championship. We created a point system. We established rules and penalties, not a fun run beer party event, not an easy mud run—a real sport!"

Warrior Dash

Mud crawling, fire leaping, extreme race from hell, worldwide locations

Launched: *2009*

Events: *50+ in 2012, 65+ planned for 2013*

Kids' Events: *None*

Minimum Age: *14*

Course Distance: *5K*

Obstacles: *12 that involve running, ducking, and climbing and will test every muscle in each competitor's body*

Terrain: *Varies by location (50 different locations)*

Signature Obstacle(s): *Warrior Roast (jumping over back-to-back fire pits) and Muddy Mayhem (a mud pit with barbed wire) finish out each event*

Hardest Obstacle: *All of the obstacles challenge each Warrior in a different way*

Gear: *Warrior Dash isn't your standard 5K race, so your outfit shouldn't be "average," either! Whether your costume is a spandex-clad superhero, medieval knight, or Smurf, take the opportunity to express your inner Warrior*

An alternative to the classic 5K, Warrior Dash is the world's largest running series and is held

> "Put down that camera and jump in, you wuss!"
> —Female participant yelling to Brett from high-low rope at Warrior Dash

on challenging and rugged terrains across the world. Participants bound over fire, trudge through mud, and scale over 12 obstacles during this fierce 5K. Warrior Dash truly is an event for all athletic abilities, from couch potatoes to novice runners to extreme athletes.

The inspiration behind Warrior Dash was to create the most bad-ass day possible. It's a day where participants can challenge themselves, be active, and get muddy. Participants tackle the course and then celebrate their accomplishments with beer, food, and live music. The unique combination of athleticism, live music, turkey legs, and beer keeps Warriors coming back for more.

Warrior Dash is partnered with St. Jude Children's Research Hospital, and encourages Warrior Dash racers to fundraise for St. Jude. With the help of 2012 participants, Warrior Dash has raised over $2 million for the hospital.

Savage Race

"The most bad-ass mud and obstacle race events," nationwide locations

Launched: *2011*

Events: *2 in 2012, 7+ in 2013*

Kids' Events: *None*

Minimum Age: *14*

Course Distance: *4–6 miles*

Obstacles: *An average of 23 giant, rugged obstacles that vary by location but may include evil monkey bars, a jump over rows of fire, a low mud crawl under barbed wire, and an ice bath*

Terrain: *Varies by location, but plan on 4–6 miles of the gnarliest terrain available*

Signature Obstacle: *Mach 7 Water Slide, which can be as tall as 45 feet—participants have reached speeds of up to 25 miles per hour*

Hardest Obstacle: *Lumberjack Lane, where participants must lug heavy objects like logs and sandbags around a long muddy loop; bad-asses are encouraged to grab two if they can*

Gear: *Athletic clothes or costumes (there's a "Most Savage Costume" contest), socks, shoes, and a kick-ass attitude*

Savage Race was founded "to create an experience unlike any other, an event that would have you questioning your sanity, an event that would absolutely kick your ass." The organizers call their participants Savages because they believe you have to find your inner barbarian to power through the race's intense four to six miles. Savage Race prides itself on having the biggest obstacles and featuring the most per mile—a true Savage challenge. It also rewards participants at the end of each race with frosty beer, sizzling barbecue, and music at the "Outrageous Savage After Party."

Savage Race's mission is to provide endurance enthusiasts with something even bigger than the race itself. It wants participants to push themselves until they think they can run no farther, climb no higher, and go no faster. Being a Savage means pushing yourself to the ultimate limit, and the high you'll feel after completing a Savage Race is something that you'll never forget.

"Most people I know come to a point in their lives where they need to prove something, either to themselves or someone else. Whether it's proof of dedication, physical, or mental strength, there's nothing quite like persevering through a challenge that once seemed impossible. I think that has been the driving force behind our success, and the growth of endurance sports as a whole."

—Sam Abbitt, founder and event manager, Savage Race

Rugged Maniac

"An Epic Day of Rugged Glory," nationwide locations

Launched: *2010*

Events: *14 in 2012*

Kids' Events: *None*

Minimum Age: *14*

Course Distance: *3.2 miles*

Obstacles: *20+*

Terrain: *"Rugged Gauntlet of Glory"—you'll figure it out!*

Signature Obstacle: *50-foot-long waterslide*

Hardest Obstacle: *12-foot-high climbing walls*

Gear: *Appropriate race clothes that are easily cleaned, like spandex pants and sports bras for girls and board shorts and fitted tops for guys*

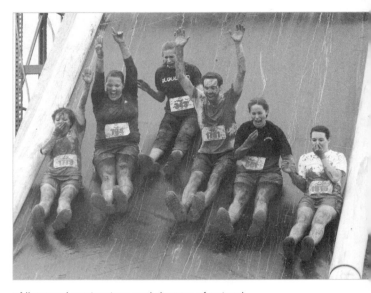

A former collegiate football player, whitewater rafting guide, and extreme skier, founder Bradford Scudder found himself trapped by the economic realities of adulthood. "I'd become a weekend warrior, every weekend was an escape from the desk. Rugged Maniac was created for people like me, to deliver an accessible day of extreme fun to those with enough heart to give it a go."

Designed with the assistance of Navy SEALs, Rugged Maniac allows people to break free from the rut of everyday life, push back their boundaries, test their physical limits, and experience what is, for many people, a life-changing day of adventure and glory. Each Rugged Maniac course features at least 20 obstacles constructed by an experienced crew of licensed contractors and dozens of natural and augmented obstacles in 3.2 miles. You'll climb over walls up to 12-feet high, crawl through mud under barbed wire, slide down a 50-foot-long water slide, jump over fire, and face many other challenges all while running through a combination of forests, fields, motocross tracks, and ski slopes. Rugged Maniac boasts the most obstacles per mile of any current event out.

"We may not be the longest—and we don't want to be. It's more about obstacles than running, and inch for inch we're the most action-packed," says Scudder. "It's all about having a good time. For some of us, that involves experimenting with our limits."

In addition to the course, Rugged Maniac offers live music, festival activities, food, and beer at its events.

Tough Mudder

**Probably the toughest event on the planet,
worldwide locations**

Launched: 2010

Events: 35 in 2012, 70 in 2013

Kids' Events: None

Minimum Age: 18

Course Distance: 10–12 miles

Obstacles: Approxmiately 29

Terrain: Varies significantly by venue; if water,
hills, or nasty terrain is present, expect to climb
over, under, or through it

Signature Obstacle: Everest, a slicked half-pipe
that participants have to scale

Hardest Obstacle: Depends on the participant

Gear: Normal running shoes (no cleats!),
lightweight clothing that dries quickly, a change
of clothes for the post party; tough, thick gloves
are optional to prevent burns from the ropes and
splinters from the walls.

Tough Mudder will push your buttons no matter your gender, shape, size, or current level of fitness. So while some Mudders are ultra-marathoners and zero-body-fat gym rats, most are regular people who are looking to take their training to the next level and have a fun time while doing it. Tough Mudder courses aren't a test of how quickly you can push yourself to the limit—the goal is to finish, and the word "race" doesn't apply. The only things to "beat" are your fears, and the only thing to "win" is a free beer. Unlike other events, Tough Mudder isn't about keeping score or time.

With over ten miles of uneven terrain, extreme temperatures, icy water, mud, and obstacles designed by British Special Forces, Tough Mudder has been dubbed "Burning Man Meets Iron Man." All participants are asked to recite the Tough Mudder pledge before starting each event, and Mudders are encouraged to

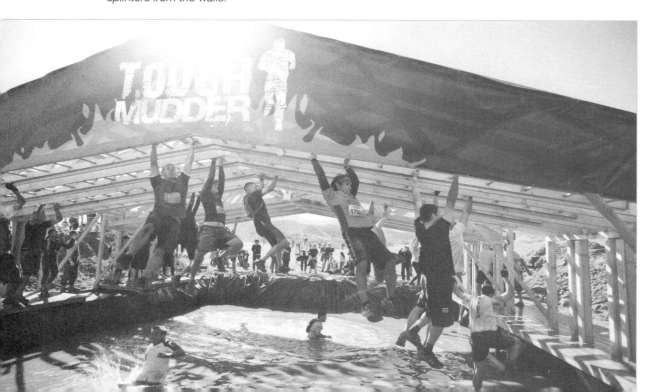

work together to dominate whatever hurdles are thrown their way, whether it's hoisting one another over a lubed-up quarter pipe or buddying up for laps in frigid water. Tough Mudders are team players who make sure no one gets left behind. But don't worry, that warm and fuzzy feeling isn't your inner stone-cold killer wimping out—it's probably the next obstacle that's been set on fire.

There are no penalties for skipping an obstacle. If plunging 15 feet into freezing cold water in Walk the Plank isn't up your alley, or running through live wires in Electroshock Therapy isn't your idea of a good time, then that's up to you—especially if you can't swim or have a heart condition. But not to fear, there are plenty of other ways to get your ass handed to you.

When Will Dean, a former counter-terrorism agent for the British government, founded Tough Mudder, he wanted to create an event that was serious about bringing the pain but didn't take itself too seriously. Camaraderie is just a big a part of the challenge as the obstacles themselves, and Mudders who want to compete in teams can help themselves to free mohawks and mullets, care of some very handy barbers at the starting line. After the event, participants can help themselves to a free beer and a chance to spring for Tough Mudder tattoos. Tough Mudder Most Respect Awards are handed out to those completing the event while overcoming illness, injury, or major life obstacles.

Tough Mudder also supports the Wounded Warrior Project and offers a $25 refund to all participants who raise $150 or more for the cause. As of this book's printing, they've raised more than $2.5 million to support the thousands of soldiers returning from the battlefield who are in need of combat stress recovery programs, adaptive sports, benefits counseling, education and employment services, and other programs that aid the healing of their mind, body, and spirit.

"By the end of 2012, we aim to replace Ironman as the preeminent brand in endurance sports."
—Alex Patterson, CMO of Tough Mudder

Alpha Warrior

**Not your typical adventure run. No miles.
No mud. No mercy. Nationwide locations**

Launched: *2013*

Kids' Events: *None*

Minimum Age: *18*

Course Distance: *Varies by location*

Obstacles: *Approximately 20*

Terrain: *Man-made modular obstacles*

Signature Obstacles: *Alcatraz, Radius Rings, Rooftops*

Hardest Obstacle: *Alcatraz, where participants encounter a 30-foot-high, multi-level obstacle testing the limits of fitness, fear, and fortitude.*

Gear/Clothing: *Athletic clothing, closed-toed shoes, and gloves are required for this course. Participants will find themselves navigating a wide range of obstacles by swinging, jumping, and crawling, requiring clothes that allow a wide range of movement.*

Consisting of a multitude of challenges varying in difficulty, size, and complexity across about 20 obstacles, Alpha Warrior is part challenge, part race, and entirely an adventure that will test your mental and physical tenacity from start to finish. Built around functional crosstraining movements, the obstacles and challenges are demanding on every muscle group in the human body and will also test your wit to adapt to the changing terrain, elevation, and obstacles in these man-made challenges. The modular obstacles each contain elements that require a blend of athletic ability, strength, and technique to pass and can be rearranged to create a new experience—more challenges, longer distances, greater heights, or even more thrilling jumps and swings—each time the course is run.

Rather than focusing on a particular running distance, the Alpha Warrior course was designed with a myriad of technical obstacles that push participants to their physical and

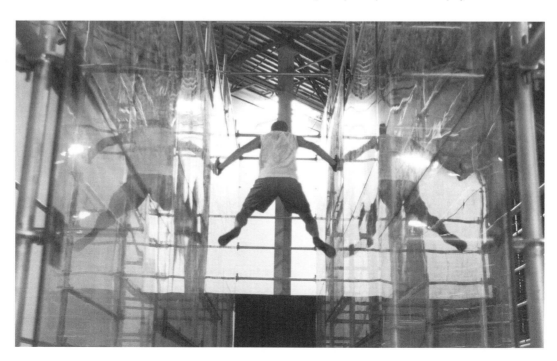

mental limit. Each modular series of obstacles was designed to feature one or more challenges that a competitor must complete or bypass to continue toward the finish. Each requires a unique skill, strength, or strategy to conquer.

Forged by an unparalleled team of athletes, architects, and engineers over the span of two years, this course was designed to challenge athletes of all ability, age, size, and gender, while featuring obstacles that do not favor any specific traditional athlete. For example, obstacles that require a balanced physique temper those who rely on upper-body strength; brute force is extremely ineffective in challenges that require technique. In other words, each cage was carefully engineered to challenge all athletes while favoring few. Whether competing as an individual or with a team, participants can expect obstacles that will amaze, impress, and be formidable barriers to completion. The elements of Alpha Warrior can be completed by many but conquered by few. Whether you're attempting to make it across the Broken Bars or flying through the air on the Rooftops, this course offers a unique opportunity to test your all-around fitness.

As one of the original Alpha Warriors that was given the opportunity to test out the course, I can tell you that it is an honor unlike any other. The massive course with towering skyscrapers of aluminum and steel evokes excitement and fear when viewing it for the first time. Immediately you realize this is nothing like you have ever seen—or been challenged by— before. The intricacies of each cage showing a limited glimpse of the challenges that you will be facing once you enter is as exhilarating as it is ominous. While the course loosely resembles a mash-up of the extremely popular TV shows *American Ninja Warrior* and *Wipeout!*, it's unique

and much more accessible to athletes of all backgrounds. Awaiting you inside each cage are barriers that require strength, agility, and guts to conquer and a proving ground for any athlete to test their limits. Think you're ready to be an Alpha Warrior? Prove it.

Alpha Warrior created the Alpha Heroes Foundation to serve military service men and women, firefighters, police officers, first responders, and any citizen who willingly puts their life at risk while serving others. All funds raised for the foundation go directly to the needs of Alpha Heroes and their families. It is the foundation's goal to address each need and wish individually in order to best serve each Alpha Hero.

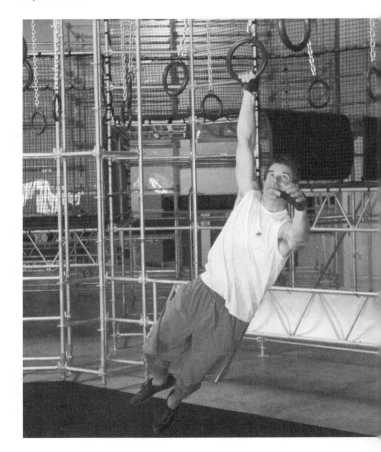

Mud Runs: Let's Get Dirty!

For the most part, you know what you're going to get out of a mud run: a fun, sloppy, messy good time. While there may be a wee bit of a challenge for some, the courses are usually created for athletes of all levels to enjoy themselves and complete the entire thing. Mud runs are a great way to get started in the world of obstacle races and bring the family along to join in the festivities. Trust me, your kids, parents, or significant other will absolutely get a huge kick out of your belly flop in the mud. Make sure to get your revenge for their snickering by giving them a big sloppy hug afterward!

Del Mar Mud Run

A 5K course in San Diego, CA, filled with military-style obstacles followed by the mud fest after-party

Launched: *2010*

Events: *1 in 2012*

Kids' Events: *None*

Minimum Age: *13*

Course Distance: *5K*

Obstacles: *Around 18 (mud pits, slides, rope swing, rope bridge, crawl tubes, monkey bars, hill climbs, tire mile, jump walls, and more)*

Terrain: *Held on the mostly flat Del Mar Fairgrounds; dirt trails, paved sections, grass, and, of course, mud*

Signature Obstacles: *9 different mud pits— Mud Pit Alpha, Bravo…all the way to Mud Pit Golf*

Hardest Obstacle: *Rope Bridge*

Gear: *Costumes, tight clothes (baggy clothes and pockets weigh you down), duct-taped shoes, a change of clothes*

Challenging yet easy enough that anyone can complete the course regardless of fitness level, the Del Mar Mud Run averages around 18 obstacles through the 3.1-mile track that winds through San Diego's historic Del Mar Fairgrounds. People gather from all over Southern California dressed in crazy costumes, ready to dive headfirst into the mud pits with their teammates. After crossing the finish line, runners celebrate with live entertainment, dancing, and free beer. There's also a large vendor village filled with food, games, and free swag. All runners receive a finisher's T-shirt, and the top individual runners and teams in each start time receive a top finisher medal.

The Challenged Athletes Foundation Operation Rebound is the official beneficiary of the run, and provides unparalleled sports opportunities and support to U.S. troops and veterans of any branch of service who've suffered permanent physical injuries. It has raised $30,000 so far through this event.

Mad Mud Run

Family-friendly fun mud run, Southwest U.S.

Launched: *2007*

Events: *4 in 2012*

Kids' Events: *MudPuppy Splash, ages 4–12*

Course Distance: *3–5 miles*

Obstacles: *Designed to fit each individual race venue, but are typical "boot camp" style—low wall, belly crawl, monkey bars, cargo net climb, hay bale obstacle, and slimy mud pit*

Terrain: *Varies significantly by venue; expect dirty trail runs and plenty of mud*

Signature Obstacle: *The Soak Zone, where kids of all ages can bring their biggest, baddest squirt guns to spray down the racers*

Hardest Obstacle: *The Mud Pit—thick, deep and gooey mud right before the finish line*

Gear: *Costumes of all types (prizes awarded) or something you're not afraid of getting trashed*

Remember back in "The History behind Ob/Mud Runs" on page 15 when we took that magical little trip through adventure races and the Camp Pendleton Mud Run? Well, it was the same journey made by Rick Eastman, which led to him creating Sierra Adventure Sports and launching Mad Mud Runs and Scavenger Dash. (Read all about Scavenger Dash on page 51).

Rick was a stockbroker with a sense of adventure that was limited to hiking and mountain biking. After watching the Eco Challenge on TV in the late '90s, he fell in love with adventure racing. "The biggest allure for me was not just the endurance aspect, but the fact that you didn't know what challenges waited for you until the race actually started," he says.

Held in Sedona, Arizona, Phoenix, Arizona, and Las Vegas, the Mad Mud Run is three to five miles of going over, under, around, and through multiple obstacles and a mud pit. You can fly solo, or grab some friends for teams of one, two, or five people. It's open to all levels of athletes.

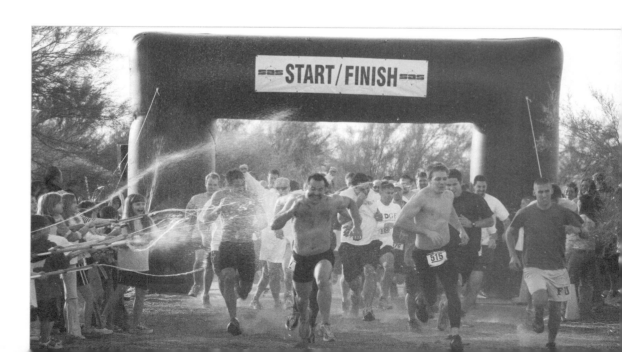

GETTIN' CHICKED

Originated in triathlons, the phrase "gettin' chicked" is a tongue-in-cheek reference to a guy getting beaten by a gal in a race. It has made its way through all forms of organized events, and it's now a source of female pride in mud runs and obstacle races. Most dudes clearly don't mind getting passed by women flying by them on the course, either—there's something quite appealing about a fit female slathered in mud as she climbs, crawls, and wriggles over obstacles, right? Yeah, that's a little sexist, but I bet there's plenty of ladies who love the muscle-bound shirtless guys running with sweat glistening on their six-packs, too. As mentioned earlier, getting muddy is hard-wired into our DNA and evokes a primal response—we're all animals after all, right?

Women have been a part of the obstacle racing scene since the beginning, although in smaller numbers than their male counterparts. Spartan Race has seen a dramatic shift in female participation over

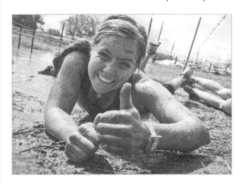

the last two years, with over 130,000 women having run an event. Over the last three years, female participation has absolutely exploded from an average of below 10% at organized events to over 30% by 2012. Road races and marathons generally have a 50/50 female-to-male split; with obstacle racing, the participation ratio is close to 40/60. That number is growing. Anecdotally, during a late afternoon heat at Warrior Dash in Florence, Arizona, over 50% of the competitors were female. This speaks volumes as to how women are embracing mud runs and taking the obstacle racing scene by storm.

Carrie Adams, founder of Rad Racing and Spartan Chicked, has been on the front lines, leading an army of women into the fray of obstacles and mud runs. She also serves as a consultant for the biggest names in obstacle races and mud runs.

"Before entering my first race I hesitated myself, but once I did it, I never looked back!" says Carrie. "It's much easier to talk a friend into running a 5K road race with you than it is to explain that there'll be fire to jump, walls to climb, buckets to carry, barbed wire to low crawl under, and technical trails to traverse!

"With the support of the Spartan Race team, I started the Spartan Chicked movement to empower women to join together and do something healthy for themselves, to ignite a fire that would keep burning long past the finish line. This network was created to educate, motivate, and empower women and girls to begin and continue active, competitive, supportive, and fitness-driven lifestyles.

"The women I've met at these races, covered head to toe in mud and scrapes that were earned on the course, have left a lasting impression on me. From new moms to grandmothers, young girls in the kids' race, cancer survivors, sisters, hardcore athletes, and first-timers alike—the energy, pride, and determination they bring to the event has brought me to tears on more than one occasion. I'm proud of what women are contributing to obstacle racing and I'm proud to be a part of such a positive force that has touched so many lives."

Women-Only Events

Not only are women an integral part of the exponential growth of mud racers worldwide, but their huge numbers have spawned a new classification of event—female-only mud runs. These events are every bit as exciting as the co-ed versions, but without all the sweaty dudes getting in the way.

LoziLu Women's Mud Run

Women-only mud run, nationwide locations

Launched: *2012*

Events: *8 in 2012*

Kids' Events: *None*

Minimum Age: *13*

Course Distance: *5K*

Obstacles: *10–12*

Terrain: *Varies depending on location*

Signature Obstacle: *Mud Bath (exfoliate and rejuvenate!)*

Hardest Obstacle: *Fishnets, 15-foot-tall cargo net climb*

Gear: *Comfy workout outfit appropriate for the weather and one you don't mind getting really dirty; team outfit and costumes are encouraged*

LoziLu (pronounced *low-ZEE-loo*) is a "Day at the Mud Spa" 5K obstacle course dedicated to providing women an experience all their own while benefiting leukemia and lymphoma research. This uniquely feminine mud run founded on fitness and fun is outfitted with a variety of optional military-ish obstacles for all fitness levels, such as Fishnets, Bad Hair Day, Tan Lines, Over It, Hot Mess, Mani-Pedi, Mud Bath, Slip & Slide, and Lost Earring. After navigating the course, pick up your bag from the valet and head to the salon for a quick Superwoman changeover. Don't forget to get your glam on and strike a pose on the red carpet after you're done with your day at the mud spa!

The idea for LoziLu emerged from the mind of a fitness-loving couple. Francis Donovan and Luisa, his then fiancée, now wife, were chatting about the best way to spread their love of fitness with the world. Having come from the elite ranks of triathlon, they knew their event had to be much more accessible than that. A mud run was perfect.

Francis and Luisa pitched their idea to their former college roommates (now also husband and wife) at the University of Wisconsin-Madison, and Team LoziLu was born. The two couples created an event that was less intimidating and had greater accessibility for all fitness levels than existing mud run events. LoziLu strives to spread happiness, health, and fitness throughout the world by leveraging the familial influence of women. It supports leukemia and lymphoma research to find a cure for blood cancers while helping cancer patients live happier lives.

Following the first LoziLu in 2012, the team received an inspirational e-mail from one of the LoziLu'ers, confirming their mission was being achieved: "I am turning 42 this summer and have fallen a bit out of shape. LoziLu has changed my life. I know that sounds silly, but I feel like I am getting younger each day! I was able to feel confident in anything I did in this run because there was no pressure!"

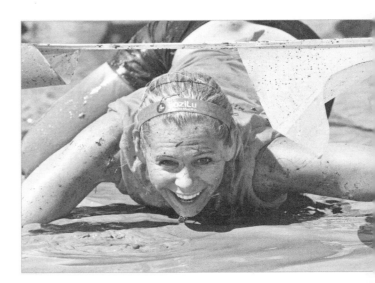

Partners/Buddies: It Takes Two

"Dude! WTF did you talk me into? See that barbed wire? That's REAL barbed wire! Look over there, that's fire—as in logs are ACTUALLY ON FIRE! What the hell is that contraption over there? Oh man, this is *bleep*-ing nuts...This. Looks. Awesome. Let's GO!"

These are the three stages of acceptance when participating in partner-based events:

1. Openly questioning your choice in friends.
2. Wondering why the hell you signed up for this crazy thing and what sadistic individual thought up this course.
3. Acceptance, giddiness, and eventually muddiness. And more giddiness.

Cahoots Duo Challenge

Two-person teamwork-required mud run and obstacle race, nationwide locations

Launched: *2011*

Events: *3 in 2012, 13 planned for 2013*

Course Distance: *3–4 miles*

Kids' Events: *None (as of publication)*

Minimum Age: *14 with parent as a partner, otherwise 18*

Obstacles: *No advance intel given on obstacles (and no course map on their website); each team will have to determine the best way to conquer an obstacle when they get to it*

Terrain: *Varies from location to location, but absolutely features some elevation change to accommodate zip lines*

Signature Obstacle: *Back to Back*

Hardest Obstacle: *Lean on Me (partners using each other to balance on suspended cables)*

Gear: *Clothes that will allow you to move unencumbered over, under, and through obstacles and that you don't mind getting really nasty; costumes are encouraged*

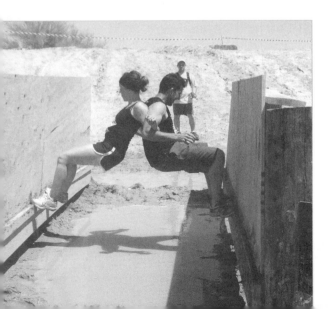

"[At Tough Guy] I remember climbing out of the water following the Death Plunge and making the comment to my buddy Joe that I didn't feel cold anymore. He noticed my lips were completely blue, my eyes were sallow, and I was shaking like crazy. He calmly stuttered through his own frozen lips, 'Th-th-that's b-because you're d-d-dying.'"

—Devon Anderson, founder,
Cahoots Duo Challenge

The obstacles you'll encounter on a Cahoots Duo Challenge course are specifically designed for you and your partner to overcome together and they get progressively more challenging as you proceed along the course. Some will be purely physical, others will have a cerebral element to them but, throughout it all, you'll have to rely on one another's strength, stamina, and grit to get through. To date, there are over two dozen obstacles that are entirely impassable without another person's assistance. Some of them even require another team to lend a few hands. There'll be zip lines, too. The best part? Each obstacle will be a surprise and you'll have no idea what to expect until you show up on race day.

In addition to the unique physical challenges, you'll encounter a handful of forks in the road, where correct passage depends on your ability to answer a question or solve a riddle. One answer leads you right, one answer leads you left. You won't know for sure whether you made the right decision or not until you've committed to a trail. If you made the wrong choice, it'll become readily apparent before too long. You'll add extra mileage to your run and more obstacles that you'd probably prefer to avoid. Consequently, each wrong turn you take has a negative impact on your "score."

Everything at Cahoots is designed to enhance the overall experience between team members, whether they're married, friends, roommates, parent/child, whatever the configuration. The goal is to make people feel like they're part of a big family. On a philosophical level, Cahoots is a call to return to the things that are important, primarily our relationships with one another.

(Learn more about Devon from Cahoots Duo Challenge on page 64 when he shares his experiences at Tough Guy.)

Scavenger Dash

"Part adventure race, part scavenger hunt, and a whole lotta fun!"; scavenger race, nationwide locations

Launched: *2009*
Events: *23 in 2012, 30+ in 2013*
Kids' Events: *None*
Minimum Age: *12*
Course Distance: *Average distance is around 5 to 8 miles by foot, but participants are allowed to use public transportation, which includes city buses and trains; in some cities (e.g., Chicago), the overall course distance can be over 12 miles*
Terrain: *Varies by location*

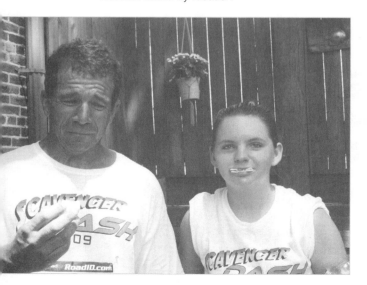

Clothing: *Whatever you'd typically wear for a day out roaming the streets; matching outfits are encouraged; comfy running/walking shoes are a good idea; cool costumes may win a prize*
Required Gear: *Digital camera (camera phones are fine, but if photos don't come out, they don't count), photo ID, $5 or more in $1 bills*
Good Idea Gear: *Cell phone, snacks, hydration backpack, GPS, city map, bus book, pens, pencils, sunblock, big hat*
Penalties: *Your bib number must be worn on the front and visible at all times or your team will be penalized 10 minutes per occurrence. Teams may only travel by foot or public transit (buses, trains, subways, ferries, trolleys); teams using any other form of transportation (taxis, hang gliders, skates, pedicabs, catching a ride, helicopter) will be immediately disqualified.*

Scavenger Dash was launched in 2009 by Rick Eastman, the founder of Sierra Adventure Sports, which also puts on the Mad Mud Run (see page 45 for more info).

In this puzzle-solving event, each two-person team is given an envelope that contains 12 clues it needs to solve. This clue sheet also serves as a passport; complete the clues, venture to the checkpoints indicated by each of the answers, and follow the instructions found there. At some points teams complete a challenge; at others they take a picture; some receive a stamp for their passport. All challenges are able to be completed by nearly anyone and teams also have the option of skipping one of the 12 clues—strategy will play a big role in which to skip. Teams may also have a mandatory clue, which will be indicated on the clue sheet.

Teams can solve clues in many ways: ask strangers, visit the library, use a smartphone or a laptop (if one of the teammates doesn't mind hauling it around). The most important resource teams can have is a great "pit crew" as their phone-a-friend. Calling someone at home who has web access can make a huge difference in solving clues.

Races may contain one or more detours, which is a choice between two challenges. Teams can choose the one they think will be fastest or the most fun. Just like on the TV show *Survivor*, teams may form alliances with other teams, if only to solve the clues. The faster teams are able solve the clues, the faster they can complete the course.

Scavenger races are all about fun, and 95% of the participants have that in mind. Some actually sign up thinking it's a bar crawl—which it's not—but the fact that it often starts and finishes in a bar lends to that understanding.

According to Scavenger Dash founder Rick Eastman, "In San Diego in 2010 we had a couple show up and start the race. The first challenge they had to overcome was to find and picture themselves with a mannequin with a head. They headed for the mall in downtown San Diego but didn't make it much farther. Upon returning to the finish line, having made it to just that single challenge, they broke out six boxes of shoes that she had found in their trip through the mall, and informed us that they'd spent most of the afternoon sipping margaritas at a local Mexican restaurant. They had a GREAT day!"

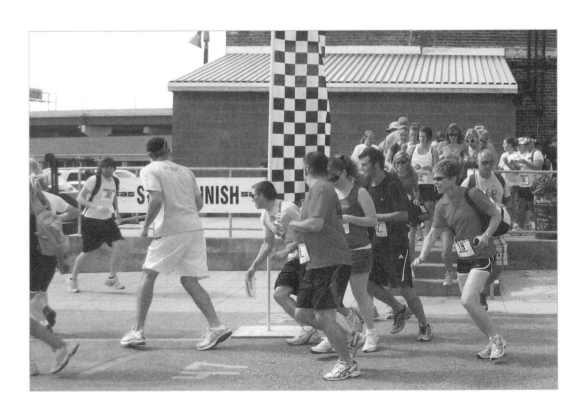

Theme-Based Events: Play Your Part in an Adventure

When I was 12 years old I wanted to be a firefighter. Well, maybe I wanted to be a cowboy or an astronaut...hell, it was three decades ago. Despite my fading memories of youth, the allure of dressing up in a costume and playing a role in an adventure still sounds pretty good to this middle-aged guy. How about you?

I won't be blasting off in an *Apollo* spacecraft anytime soon (although Sir Richard Branson may have something to say about that) but I can sign up for a theme-based event and be transformed into a hero rushing into a burning building to save a damsel in distress, the protagonist struggling to escape a crumbling town as the apocalypse rains destruction all over the planet, or the leading man in a B movie being chased by flesh-eating undead. If I'm feeling rather randy, I can even slip beneath the squirmy skin of a zombie and join their war against the living in a quest for brains. Who says you can't act like a kid and play make-believe?

Obstacle Apocalypse

Athletic adventure where you attempt to escape the course before time runs out, nationwide locations

Launched: 2011

Events: 2 in 2012, 8+ in 2013

Kids' Events: None

Minimum Age: 18

Course Distance: 5K

Obstacles: 27+

Terrain: Varies by location

Signature Obstacle: Paintball Target Practice—a successful shot earns you a shortcut

Hardest Obstacle: Getting an egg over a cargo net in one piece

Gear: Athletic gear that will allow you to run, climb, carry stuff, and survive

Do you have the speed, strength, agility, and intelligence necessary to survive the coming apocalypse? Obstacle Apocalypse is all about expanding on the idea of what an athletic adventure race can be with *Amazing Race*–type tasks and humor all set within a basic theme of escaping all the elements of an apocalypse before time runs out.

Obstacle Apocalypse courses are broken down into three sections:

The Beginning of the Apocalypse: Racers must navigate smoke, fire, fallen logs, and debris.

Escape the Burning Town: Adventurers are forced to climb over/under/through a fallen building, and grab something and drag it over an obstacle in order to make it out alive.

Survive the Apocalypse: To survive the final stage in time, contestants must swim, run, and even crawl to the...Oktoberfest after-party!

Sense of humor? Check. "Think fast, run faster" is one of their mottos, while "Run now, beer later" could easily be another. Runners also get to pick their own way to enjoy the day, including choosing alternate routes, jamming to deejayed tunes along the course, and even a polka band rocking the Octoberfest party at the finish line.

Hero Rush

Firefighter-themed obstacle race and experience, nationwide locations

Launched: *2011*

Events: *11 in 2012, 22+ in 2013*

Kids' Events: *Mini Heroes Firefighter Adventure Course, ages 4–6; Junior Heroes Firefighter Adventure Course, ages 7–13*

Minimum Age: *14*

Course Distance: *5K*

Obstacles: *20+*

Terrain: *Varies based on location, but centered around the "Inferno Midway" with obstacles and barriers of all shapes and sizes that firefighters routinely have to navigate*

Signature Obstacle: *Towering Inferno*

Hardest Obstacle: *Basement Entrapped*

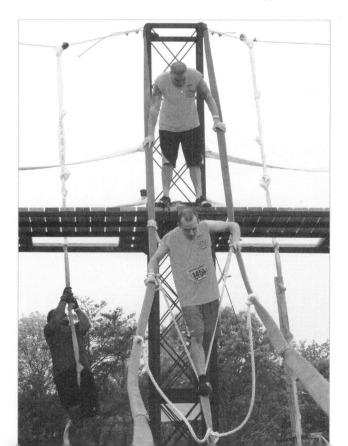

Gear: *Comfortable clothing that you don't mind getting dirty, wet, and potentially soot-stained, as well as clothing that inspires you (if you're fire/EMS, wear your department shirt; if you're military, wear your unit shirt; etc.); solid running shoes or other sturdy, appropriate footwear*

Hero Rush is all about experiencing the life of a firefighter. You'll run an intense 5K+ race with multiple fire-related obstacles: climb ladders and slide down poles, crawl through windows and break down doors, scramble through HAZMAT slime and locate trapped victims. But be careful—you might get the fire hoses turned on you! Every obstacle simulates a real scenario a firefighter might face. For example, "Towering Inferno" is modeled after actions taken in a high-rise building fire, where the water from floors above will rain down on those working below as they try to climb higher and fight the fire; from the platform at the top, racers plunge down a 20-foot waterslide to a small pool below. "Basement Entrapped" simulates what happens when a staircase collapses and a firefighter is trapped with no way out. To complete this obstacle, participants climb to a 20-foot platform by way of a knotted fire hose; from the top, they must navigate a rope bridge made of fire hoses, one to balance on as they walk and two above to hold onto.

With nearly 30 combined years as firefighters, Dave Iannone and Christopher Hebert conceived this wicked firefighter-themed obstacle race. Hero Rush brings the theme full circle by partnering with fire-service charities that benefit from race fees and donations, inviting local fire departments to come out and participate with the community, and creating an atmosphere that invites everyone to celebrate the hero within.

Run for Your Lives

Zombie-themed obstacle race, mud run, and fight for your life, North American locations

Launched: 2011

Events: 13 in 2012, 25+ in 2013

Course Distance: 5K

Kids' Events: None

Minimum Age: 14

Obstacles: Approximately 10–12 man-made and natural obstacles

Terrain: Trails, mud, blood, and obstacles/structures to go over, under, or through; multiple routes to reach the finish line

Signature Obstacle: Blood Pit

Hardest Obstacle: Staying Alive

Penalties: If a runner loses all of the flags on their flag belt, they're no longer eligible for prizes

Gear: Zombie repellent; active clothes that'll let you run, climb, and slog through mud and that you don't mind tossing in the trash afterward

Fans of AMC's *The Walking Dead*, Run for Your Lives creators Ryan Hogan and Derrick Smith provide people with a one-of-a-kind experience, and they do so by keeping as many race details as possible tightly under wraps. This breeds fear and uncertainty in the minds of each racer—just how zombies like it! No one should have the benefit of knowing what horrific things may lie ahead.

Each race takes participants through a series of manmade and natural obstacles over a 5K zombie-infested course. They're physically challenging but not impossible; plan on mud, water, and maybe some blood. Racers will need to climb, crawl, duck, and dive their way to the finish line, all with a bunch of flesh-starved undead on their tail.

Racers, each wearing a flag football-like belt with three flags, must make strategic choices to find the quickest route to the finish line with at least one flag to remaining to complete the race as a survivor. Choose wisely, or the 5K might turn into a 10K.

In another gruesome twist, Run For Your Lives lets you choose what side you're on: flesh-eating zombie or fresh-meat runner. Zombies are given professional make-up, tattered clothes, and zombie training lessons so they can safely pull runners' flags. Survivors and newly created "zombies" (those who finish without flags) are able to celebrate at the Apocalypse Party, a post-race event that features live, local entertainment, music, vendors, food, beverages, and, of course, zombies.

ROC (Ridiculous Obstacle Challenge)

5K obstacle course filled with ridiculous and epic obstacles, San Diego, CA

Launched: *2011*

Events: *1 in 2012*

Kids' Events: *None*

Minimum Age: *13*

Obstacles: *10+*

Terrain: *Natural, manmade, and completely ridiculous*

Course Distance: *5K*

Signature Obstacle: *Wrecking Ball*

Most Difficult Obstacle: *Wrecking Ball*

Gear: *Ridiculous costumes*

This 3.1-mile course features the world's largest inflatable slide and an obstacle that actually fights back: a floating string of barrels over a pool of water that racers must navigate while swinging wrecking balls fly from all directions trying knock them off. Other obstacles include a wrecking ball (just try making it across without getting knocked into the water), a rope swing, crawl tubes, monkey bars, hill climbs, tight rope traverse, slip 'n' slides, and tire mile.

During the ROC race, you'll also see some of the most ridiculous outfits, costumes, and characters ever. After crossing the finish line, runners stick around for the after-party, with live entertainment, free beer garden, games, food and more. All runners receive a high-quality finisher's T-shirt, and the top individual runners and teams in each start time receive a top finisher's medal.

The Challenged Athletes Foundation (CAF) Operation Rebound is the official beneficiary of the run. CAF Operation Rebound provides unparalleled sports opportunities and support to U.S. troops and veterans of any branch of service who have suffered permanent physical injuries. ROC has raised $30,000 so far.

Events for the Kids

Remember when you were a kid? A old tire on a rope was good for a few hours of fun, and if you were from my neighborhood you soon learned how to dive through or do backflips off of it. Building ramps to jump off with our bikes was the first thing we did after coming home from school and we kept piling cinder blocks (or the youngest neighbors) to jump over until Mom turned the porch light on. We weren't nuts—that's what being a kid in the 1970s was like. Today, ehhh...not so much.

For as much as we've advanced in the last 40 years in technology, it seems we've lost touch with the fun and excitement that comes with being a kid and attempting some off-the-wall stuff that would never fly today (like "ghost riding" your bike down a hill or any attempt to defy gravity using bungee cords). I distinctly remember an entire summer spent wallowing in mud puddles, chasing lizards around the swamp, and running from some deranged lunatic with a caddle prod. Then again, that may have been one of the times my parents forgot me at the zoo.

Luckily, there's a solution to the "play dates" and hand sanitizer that whippersnappers today have grown up with. A bunch of events feature a kid's version and, let's face it—where there's mud, you'll usually find a kid. Here's an interesting dichotomy: Most competitors run a whole race while dreading the mud pit at the end, while to most kids that bog of murkiness is like their own little nirvana.

Want to know if an event is kid-friendly? Our site www.mudrunguide.com lists whether each race has an event just for the little ones or not. If it does and you're competing in the adult version, remember to pack some extra towels and dry clothes for your kids; they may have to wait around after finishing their race for you to compete. As far as kid's gear goes, it's a good recommendation to make sure their outfit covers elbows and knees if you'd like to prevent a few extra boo-boos. A sure-fire tip to save you a few hours at bath time is to use some form of earplug that will keep mud out; many a racer has dislodged a wad of mud days after an event with a cotton swab. Check out the "Gear Guide" on page 26 for more tips on adult gear; you just may get some good ideas for the kids, too.

Here is just a sample of events for kids, as well as a nationwide "boot camp" built on the obstacle race template. In no way is this an all-inclusive list as events change daily.

Bounce Boot Camp

Outdoor inflatable obstacle course & fitness training for kids 5–14, nationwide franchises
Launched: 2011
Events: Weekly kids' fitness classes
Course Distance: Varies by class, 1-hour duration
Obstacles: Cones, balls, agility ladders, hurdles, battle ropes, etc.
Signature Obstacle: General Jumper
Hardest Obstacle: Battle Ropes
Gear: Athletic clothes; socks or bare feet on the inflatables

Bounce Boot Camp is the first obstacle course–style fitness program utilizing inflatable castles, slides, obstacle courses, and other interactive equipment. Thomas Hill and his team have developed the course to include leadership training, nutritional counseling, strength building, and cardiovascular conditioning so that kids can get fit, develop athletic skill, flexibility, dexterity, agility, endurance, and have fun—all while learning life lessons and developmental skills to be future leaders.

Centered around their custom-made inflatable equipment, including the General Jumper, classes implement other equipment such as cones, balls, hurdles, quick foot ladders, and the signature Battle Ropes. Each class is set up differently, providing an element of surprise and excitement as well as teaching kids how to adapt to new challenges. After warm-ups and instructions, the kids are divided into groups and are led by the Generals to face off against the course. Every ten minutes, the groups rotate to a new series of challenges until all stations are complete. The Finisher awaits the kids once they're done with their training; each child runs through the entire obstacle course, engaging each station, competing against the clock, their friends, or for just some good-natured fun and exercise.

The goal of Bounce Boot Camp is to teach kids that tackling challenges and solving obstacle courses can be fun and a great way to get fit. These types of activities can also provide them with healthy habits they can use for a lifetime. To find a Bounce Boot Camp near you, check out www.mudrunguide.com/bouncebootcamp.

Kids Fit Jr. Spartan Adventure (Spartan Race)

Jr. Spartan | Ages 4–9, 1/2 mile
Varsity Spartan | Ages 10–13, 1 mile

Spartan Race is not only limited to adult fun— kids can participate in their very own Spartan Race with a variety of scaled-down obstacles and their own mini festival area filled with games and children's challenges. The Jr. Spartan Adventure (ages 4–9) is half a mile, while the Varsity Spartan Adventure (ages 10–13) is 1 mile. The mission is to inspire children to develop a love for fitness at an early age.

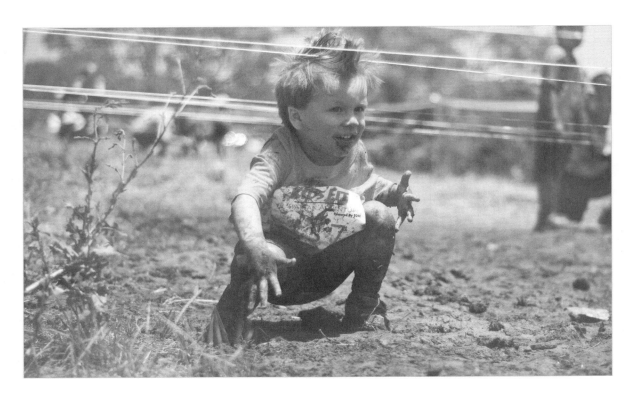

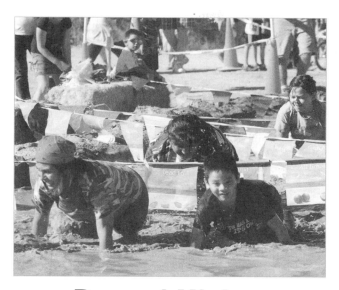

Rugged Mini-ac (Rugged Maniac)

Rugged Maniac's kid's course is built for children ages 3–8 who want to run through mud, climb over tires, and jump over walls. Not every Rugged Maniac race will have a Mini-ac course, so please check the individual event facts beforehand. Older children can run it but it won't be much of a challenge for them. Events that do not feature a Mini-ac course will have other forms of entertainment (such as bounce houses) available for children.

Screwball (T).H.U.G (Tough Guy)

Screwball (T).H.U.G is an event for kids between 10 and 16 who are accompanied by an adult. Kids/'tweens/teens will need every last ounce of mental and physical strength they can muster to rise to this challenge.

MudPuppy Splash (Mad Mud Run)

During the Mad Mud Run races, kids can participate by spraying down Mom and Dad with big squirt guns in the Splash Zone. Immediately after the last adult finishes, the MudPuppy Splash opens up to 4- to 12-year-olds, with simple obstacles to tackle before jumping into the mud pit. The course is 100 meters in Phoenix, 200 meters in Las Vegas, and 300 meters in Sedona.

Hero Rush

There are two kid's courses at Hero Rush. The Mini Heroes Course is a short dash for the 4–6 crowd that's completely free, and it runs on a regular schedule throughout the event. The Junior Heroes Course is a 1/2 mile with smaller obstacles for those ages 7–13. These fun courses will also teach kids a thing or two about fire safety.

Extreme: Only the Strongest Will Survive

You're not worthy. Well, unless you're the best of the best at obstacle racing, you're not worthy of toeing the line at these events…yet. Can you get there? Absolutely. The invitation is wide open to those who are willing to put in the hard work and practice, train, and race their ass off to get to the top of this sport. These events are invite-only or only the toughest SOBs need apply. Tough Guy may be the easiest of the list to get into as they feature two yearly events (a double-length version in the summer and a brutally cold event in the winter) and don't have a qualifying system like Spartan Ultra Beast and Toughest Mudder do—you just need to be nuts enough to sign up.

Spartan Ultra Beast

Ultimate Spartan Race course, marathon-distance, Killington, VT

Launched: 2012

Events: 1

Qualifying: Submit your race resume and three sentences why you belong in the race

Course Distance: 26.2 miles

Obstacles: Dozens of the hardest obstacles Spartan Race has to offer

Terrain: Brutal trails, hills, and mud at one of the largest ski areas in Vermont

Gear: Competitors are on their own against the terrain and elements, plus there's an outside chance of snow and ice; be prepared

Spartan Ultra Beast is a 26.2-mile Obstacle Race from Hell. If you've done any race anywhere in the world, whether a mud run, fun run, Olympic run, bike race, death march, or any kind of event claiming to be the "toughest race on the planet," you'll be happy to know that the Spartan Ultra Beast is where it ends. This is the world's first marathon-distance obstacle race. Elite racers confront two loops of the main course before finding the finish line. For everyone's safety and for the competitive nature of the event, competitors must apply for acceptance in the Ultra Beast marathon. Hopefuls are required to send an e-mail to the race directors with their race resume accompanied by a three-sentence description of why they should be chosen to participate in the event.

> "You ran a marathon? Now, isn't that cute…"
> —Joe DeSena, co-founder, Spartan Race

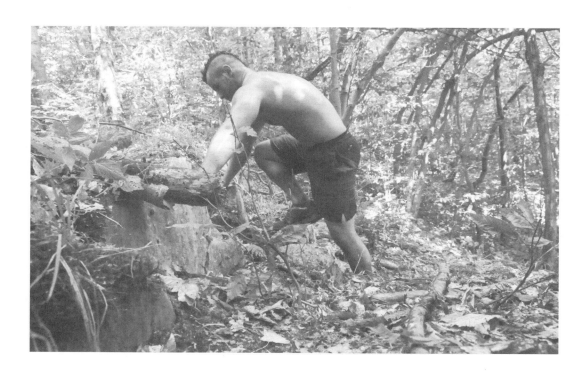

Tough Guy

A real-time battlefield experience, Perton, Staffordshire, England

Launched: *1987*

Events: *2 in 2012 (January Winter Survival and July Nettle Warrior)*

Qualifying: *Having the guts to sign up and travel to Staffordshire to compete*

Kid's Event: *Yes, (T).H.U.G., ages 10–16*

Minimum Age: *16*

Course Distance: *9–12 miles*

Obstacles: *25+*

Terrain: *Challenging, hilly trail, the "Killing Fields"*

"Welcome to Tough Guy, the safest most dangerous event in the world!" Developed by the dastardly mind of Billy Wilson, a.k.a. Mr. Mouse, over 25 years ago, Tough Guy is commonly referred to as "the world's most demanding one-day survival ordeal" or "the toughest race in the world," as the nearly 30% failure-to-finish rate of competitors serves to prove. While Mr. Mouse offers a 19K race each summer that features two loops through the "Killing Fields," the "January Winter Survival" on the same grounds must be completed for competitors to be considered a real Tough Guy finisher.

Held during the icy grip of winter in Staffordshire, England, Tough Guy is as much a battle against the elements as it is a fight to conquer the countless "man-made assaults for individual challenge" that litter the Killing Fields. But first, racers must survive the convivial-sounding Country Miles, which start with a climb up slick and muddy Trample Hill and continue with fences, ditches, cargo nets, and a hillside slalom. Each frozen mud pit greets the shins of the racers with shards of ice, forcing them to trudge forward beyond their pain thresholds to the next obstacle.

The Killing Fields begin with the menacing Tiger: a climb up a 40-foot A-frame followed by a run through electrified wires with shocks that can bring adults to their knees. Walls, ropes, barbed wire, mud, tires, and fire are but a prelude to the horror of the Vietcong Torture Chamber Tunnels or Underwater Tunnels. Here, racers claw for an overhead opening to breathe from while submerged in the freezing cold, murky water. The fear of drowning coupled with the brain-stopping cold water proves too much for as many as 25% of racers. Those who continue have more than a dozen more sadistic barriers between them and the finish: Tough Guy glory and a cup of hot chocolate.

World's Toughest Mudder

The 24-hour culminating event of the yearly Tough Mudder calendar, Englishtown, NJ

Launched: *2011*

Events: *1*

Qualifying: *1000 spots, limited to top 5% of Tough Mudder finishers based on submitted time or drawn from a wildcard lottery.*

Course Distance: *Continual laps of an 8–10 mile course for 24 hours*

Obstacles: *"A healthy dose"*

Terrain: *Trails, mud, water, ice, mayhem, and misery*

Gear: *Racers are allowed to pitch their tent in the pit area and sleep, eat, or do whatever they need to do during the course of the 24-hour race.*

For those who are in it for cash and glory, Tough Mudder puts together a once-a-year event for the top 5% of racers. World's Toughest Mudder takes the concept of being a Tough Mudder to a whole new level. This extreme competition puts the world's most hardcore Mudders through a grueling 24-hour challenge designed to find the toughest man, woman, and four-person team on the planet. When the mud settles on November 18th, a select few winners will have bested 500,000 other Mudders worldwide for the right to call themselves the World's Toughest Mudders.

Competitors have 24 hours to complete as many laps of a Tough Mudder course on steroids as they can. At the 24-hour mark, all competitors must complete the lap they are on and the winners will be whichever participants have completed the greatest number of laps in the allotted 24+ hours. In the event that multiple participants complete the winner's total number of laps, the winners will be whichever participants cross the finish line of the final lap first.

Unlike other Tough Mudder events, this event is a competition and the winners will receive cash prizes of $15,000 (male and female individual winners) and $20,000 (team winners). Participants will be required to wear timing chips and are subject to the event's official rules. That said, participants are strongly encouraged to embody the Mudder spirit of teamwork and camaraderie to help each other through the course.

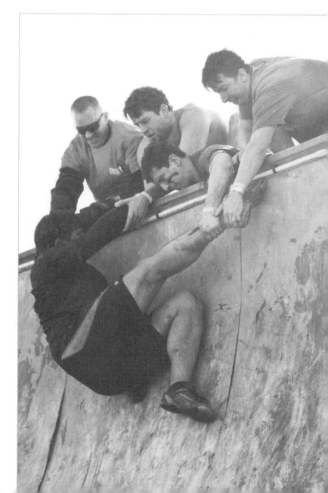

Death Race

Invite-only extremely demanding obstacle race with mental and physical challenges, Pittsfield, VT

Founded: *2004*

Events: *1*

Qualifying: *Extreme mental fortitude, online registration at www.youmaydie.com*

Course Distance: *Varies in mileage and time; finish is when co-founders Andy and Joe decide the race is over*

Obstacles: *Mental and physical*

Terrain: *Hilly, rugged Vermont mountain trails with water crossings; extremely difficult*

Signature Obstacle: *Mental torture, "Death Race Mindf*ck" (as they like to call it)*

Hardest Obstacle: *Surviving to finish the race*

Gear: *Events last longer than 24 hours, so layers that allow you to move freely are most likely a good idea, as is well-fitting footwear that can handle trails replete with rocks, mud, and water crossings to minimize blisters*

Death Race is different than any other event; it emulates life. While every other event is designed for you to finish, with aid stations, directions, volunteers giving you a pat on the back and cheering you on, this one is completely designed to break people physically and mentally. Death Race doesn't tell you when the race is going to start, when it'll end, how long it'll be, what to wear, bring, eat—it's designed to be just like life. There are no set answers and you have no idea what you're doing until you get there.

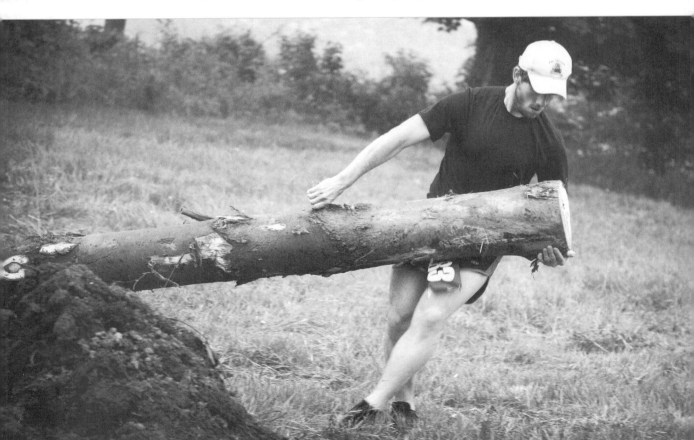

Each event has a theme that goes so much deeper than just banners or e-mails with gladiator photos; they're diabolically chosen to make you question yourself, your priorities, and everything about your life. The wrong choices may even kill you. Death Race starts the minute you sign up, months before the event. The uncertainty will consume you, enrage you, and get in your head to knock you off your game. Death Race will piss you off weeks before the gun goes off.

Says cofounder Joe DeSena, "The few individuals who can keep their mind clear and focused while continuing to progress forward fare considerably better than the average individual. The elite of this group are the ones who complete the event and inspire others—including everyone here at Death Race. We created the race to find these superheroes, and it's a life-altering event for everyone involved when they realize their full potential. If I find one superhero per race, then I consider it a rousing success."

A very large percentage of racers are repeat offenders; Death Race gets under their skin and becomes a part of them. For the 80% or so that don't finish, those with the drive and determination to complete the race are sucked back in to submit their entry request for the following year, knowing full well the race will be entirely different in length of time, distance covered, obstacles, and theme.

During the 2010 Death Race, entrants were forced to look inside themselves for their view on greed and what money truly meant to them by carrying $50 dollars along with them and making decisions on how or where they should spend their money—should they donate it, use it to buy safe passage around obstacles, purchase items

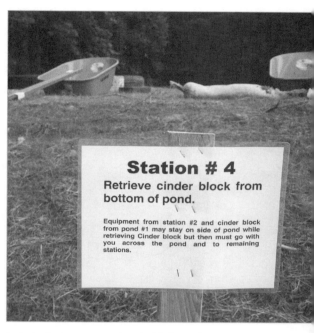

Station # 4
Retrieve cinder block from bottom of pond.

Equipment from station #2 and cinder block from pond #1 may stay on side of pond while retrieving Cinder block but then must go with you across the pond and to remaining stations.

to help their quest, or horde it? Sounds simple enough, only it wasn't a 50 dollar bill or even 50 singles, but 5000 pennies they had to carry in backpacks, weighing in at over 34 pounds. Each participant chose his/her own way to use the money, and one nearly paid the price with his life. Weighed down by over 30 pounds of zinc and copper, this competitor was dragged under the water by his backpack. Had it not been for other racers, he may have drowned.

Not only are the elements constantly changing, but also is the duration. As of 2012, the longest Death Race clocked in at a whopping 70 hours, while the shortest to date was completed in 12 hours. During the latter event, Joe was a competitor and his partners engineered the course. Upon finishing it in 12 hours, he deemed that event was "too soft" and made the decision on the spot that no racer would ever walk off any of his courses in the future and utter that phrase.

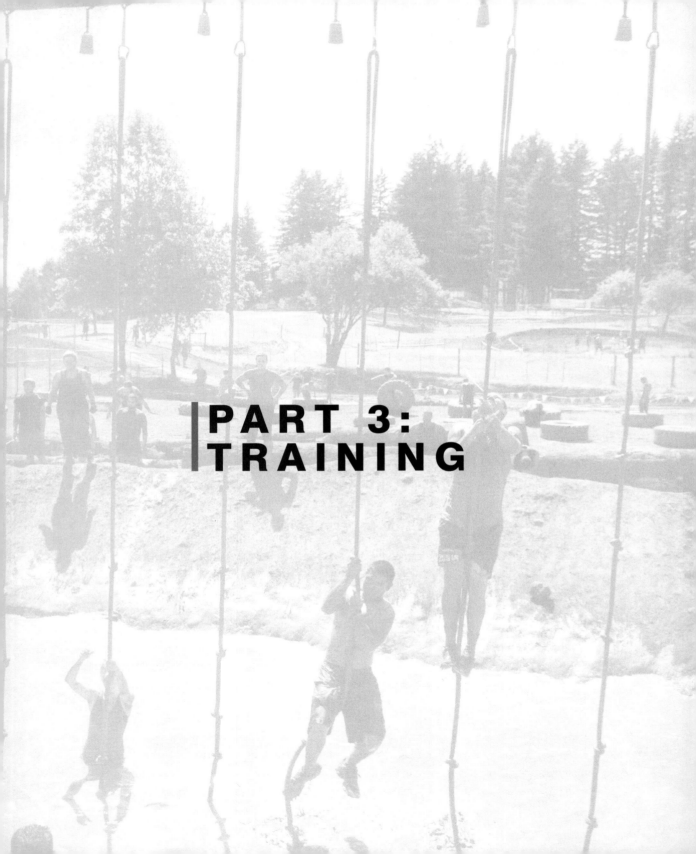

PART 3: TRAINING

Prepare to Dominate All Obstacles

Back on pages 14 and 32 I listed about 50 different nasty little surprises that are waiting for everyone in some form or fashion on nearly every course. With the boundless creativity (some call it masochistic tendencies) of race directors and course builders at these events, newer, harder, and more complicated barriers are erected each time a race comes to town. You'll never be prepared for every last one, but the list in this section covers a lot of the basic ones that you'll see so you can be prepared for those.

The first time you'll see most obstacles is on the course, unless you've built an eight-foot wall in your backyard or spent an afternoon at the local skate park trying to climb up the half pipe—but you absolutely should do both if you can (instructions for creating your own wall for less than $200 can be found on our website).

Your house, yard, and neighborhood (especially playgrounds) are full of stuff to practice obstacle training. Who says they're for kids only? As long as the stuff will hold your weight,[3] there's no reason you can't climb, swing, or crawl under and over any of it to prepare your body for the stuff you'll see on race day. Actually, I'm counting on it! Consider this your permission to act like a kid. Who cares if the neighbors gawk—you're developing your inner bad-ass!

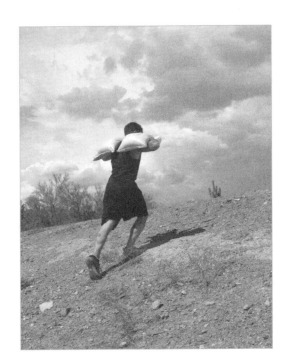

I've broken down each of the most common obstacles you'll find on race day into three categories and developed specific workouts for each based on the types of movements, strength, or ability you'll need to conquer:

The **Strength Workout** is all about pushing, pulling, and lifting stuff. Flipping tractor tires, carrying sandbags, and dragging blocks of concrete with a rope all fall into this category.

The **Dexterity Workout** is dedicated to getting your body over, under, and through obstacles on the course. Walls, cargo nets, and ropes all challenge your technique even more than brute strength. This workout will help you plan your attack.

The **Speed & Endurance Workout** will help you develop the speed and endurance to torch the course between obstacles. On race day you'll run through water, mud, and fire, up and down hilly trails, and across terrain of all types. This workout will help you get through them all more quickly than you ever thought possible.

---

3 Seriously, make sure anything you're planning to climb on or swing from will support at least twice your bodyweight before you do anything that'll destroy property or hurt yourself or any combination of both. It's on you to test out and make sure first. Don't put yourself or others in danger. The point is to get stronger, build your confidence, and have fun—not break, tear, or rupture anything.

Strength Workout:
Moving Stuff

The good news about the "Moving Stuff" category is that you can train and practice these moves with nearly an exact replica of the items you'll be dealing with out on the course. The bad news is it's going to be a tough-as-hell workout on your whole body. You'll be moving around heavy and awkward objects in order to develop the strength, technique, and confidence you need to tackle these nefarious little bastards come race day.

OBSTACLE TO DOMINATE
Weighted Carry

"Ladies grab one. Guys get two. Bad-asses pick up three." – Sign at Arizona Super Spartan Race

This challenge is pretty straightforward: Pick up something heavy from one place and carry it to the designated point, often right back where you started. The object to be carried can be a sandbag, log, bucket of sand, rocks, concrete blocks…or anything that's light enough for you to lift and carry yet heavy enough to make your arms, legs, and core scream for mercy after a few minutes. Hills and other obstacles are often thrown in to add to the misery. To prepare for this, you'll need to develop your full body strength by performing nearly identical tasks with some heavy items you can find around the house or at a local hardware store.

CREATE YOUR OWN WEIGHTS TO CARRY

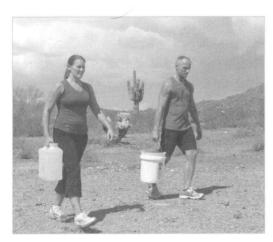

Beginners can start with a gallon jug of water at just under 8.5 pounds. These make a perfect, extremely inexpensive weight for all of the exercises in this category, and you can even use it to hydrate between sets. Once you've mastered the weight of water, dump it out and add some sand. Depending on density, you can easily double the weight. Keep in mind that the handle may need some reinforcement. Can you say duct tape?

Most big hardware stores or nurseries carry bags of sand. Look for a 40-pound version in a tear-resistant bag; these are usually the types of sandbags that are designed for ballast and not what you'd purchase to fill a kid's sandbox. If it comes with a built-in handle that's fine, but in order to build your grip strength, you'll alternate between using it and not. Your local fire department may also be able to provide some sandbags; they probably won't charge you, so feel free to make a little donation. If you'd rather make your own, a heavy garbage bag and some duct tape will be an inelegant yet workable short-term solution and also allow you to select a weight that'll work best for you. Dump as much sand as you'd like into a bag and form it into the rounded rectangular shape of a sandbag. Leave a little room for the sand to shift inside; this'll make your stabilizer muscles work even harder to steady yourself when the load moves as you shift the bag or walk. Wrap the bag as many times as you can, trim the excess, and wrap it all up with duct tape.

A 5-gallon bucket is one of the easiest items to come by, and you can pick them up at a hardware or paint store for as little as $5. Add some water, sand, or rocks and you have a weighted object with a handle. Speaking of handles, to build your grip strength, increase the thickness of your bucket's handle with duct tape or simply wrap a towel around it to really force your forearms and fingers to work harder.

Sandbag Carry

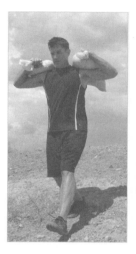
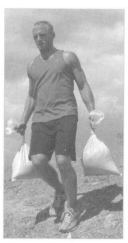

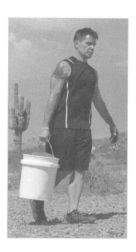

This one is simple. For either time or distance, lift and carry a sandbag (or two). Hug it against your chest like a teddy bear, cradle it like a baby, plop it on your shoulder, and grasp it down at your side like a bag of loot. No matter what you chose, the goal of this exercise is to add significantly to your body weight and force you to figure out how to carry a load and still continue to move forward, up, over, through, or around barriers. Time yourself: Go as far as you can or do repeated climbs up a hill. No matter your goal, you'll be working your entire body to hold the shifting weight with this simple and effective exercise. If you have to take the dog for a walk, bring along "Sandy," too!

SPECIFIC WEIGHTED CARRY EXERCISES

SINGLE-HAND FARMER'S WALK

Although not much different from the side "bag-of-loot" grip in the sandbag carry, the farmer's walk is a specific discipline that's a great full-body workout. This single-armed variety is excellent for developing stability by promoting instability with weights.

With one weighted bucket at your side, squat down and grasp the handle with your palm facing your leg. Drive through your heels and lift the bucket up while straightening your legs. Engage your core muscles to keep your spine straight and your body vertical. If you're unable stay erect and are leaning toward the side of your body where the bucket is, lower the bucket and remove some weight.

With the bucket raised, walk forward slowly for the time or distance outlined in Strength Workout and then place the bucket on the ground, swap hands, and repeat.

OVERHEAD WEIGHTED WALK

Yes, this is as easy as it sounds—you lift a weight over your head and walk slowly. It's also a great way to activate and strengthen core and stabilizer muscles, as well as work your arms and legs. This exercise can be performed with a weight, medicine ball, rock, or log. Just

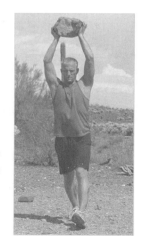

be extremely careful you don't drop it on your head (or toes).

Stand with your feet about hip-width apart and raise the weight over your head. Extend your arms straight overhead with your elbows just slightly bent and not locked. Engage your core as if you were about to be hit in the stomach with a tennis ball; try not to arch your back.

Keeping your back tall and straight, walk for the targeted amount of time or steps. Then lower the weight to chest height, squat down, and place it on the ground between your feet.

Tractor Tire Flip

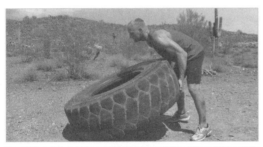

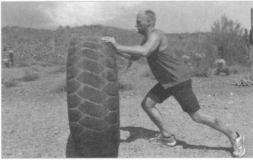

Why on earth would anyone in their right mind decide that flipping tractor tires was a good idea? Well, mostly because they look really intimidating, provide a sizeable challenge, and all in all are actually kind of fun to flip. Who would've thought that those old tractor tires that

farmers couldn't wait to get rid of from behind their barns would become such a sought-after item thanks to obstacle races? This maneuver will require a nice deep squat for you to place your hands properly, a strong drive from your legs, core, and upper body to get it moving, and an explosive burst to get the tire past vertical and flipped over.

Finding a used tractor tire may be simple or difficult depending on where you live. If you can track one down that's medium-sized from a tire store, they might actually be happy to give it away (you're saving them the recycling costs) and all you'll need to do is pick it up and get it home. This isn't necessarily an easy task, though. These tires weigh 400 to 600 pounds and will require at least a few helpers to load and unload them from a pickup truck bed. When you're searching through the tire pile, pick one that you can flip over based on the exercise description below. It makes no sense to drag home a monster and end up hurting yourself. You can always go back and pick up a heavier one later, and the tire shop workers will most likely be impressed with your tenacity!

Tractor Tire Flip

Getting a tire is the best way to prepare you for the real obstacle, but it may be too difficult for beginners. If you're new to this type of exercise, start with Squat & Toss and Band Squat & Press first and work your way up to the big tire.

Place your feet wider than your shoulders with your toes pointed outward a bit and up against or under the edge of the tire; you want to be as close as possible to the edge of the tire to minimize the reach forward and accompanying stress on your lower back. Place your hands palms-up under the tire as far as you can. You may not have a good hand position to start because of the tire's position and will have to readjust slightly once you get the tire up and in motion.

Squat straight down, lean forward slightly, place your chest on the tire (if it's a thin tire, your chest may be as much as a foot above the tire's edge), and transfer your weight to the balls of your feet. The lift is an explosive move—you'll simultaneously push 90% upward and 10% forward from the balls of your feet while lifting the tire using your hips, arms, and chest. Push your hips forward rapidly to extend your legs and drive the tire upward.

When the tire is about 45 degrees, shift your hands to an overhand grip, step forward with your dominant leg, and use your momentum to push the tire completely over. *If you lose momentum, get stuck, or can't complete the lift, jump backward out of the way of the falling tire.*

Even if you were unable to complete the flip, developing your strength in the first portion of the lift is the most important. With repeated effort and work on your technique, you'll figure it out.

SPECIFIC TIRE FLIP EXERCISES

SQUAT & TOSS

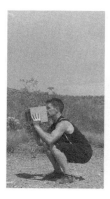 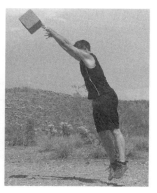

No tire? No problem! You can use a medicine ball, rock, log, or nearly any weighted object that you can throw to mimic the tire flip. Start light while you're learning the movement; you can always add more weight as you go along. Pay careful attention to lower back pain; if it hurts, you're putting too much stress on that area through bad form. Drop down in weight and use a basketball to get the move right and perform it painlessly.

Note: You're going to be throwing something heavy, so make sure you're outside and can't break anything, anyone else, or yourself. Be creative in the objects you use, but be smart and safe first.

Place the object that you'll be tossing on the ground and stand with your feet on either side of it slightly wider than your shoulders and your toes pointed slightly outward.

Squat straight down and reach under the object with both hands, shifting your weight slightly forward to the balls of your feet.

The lift is an explosive move—you'll simultaneously push 90% upward and 10% forward from the balls of your feet while lifting the object using your hips, arms, and chest. Push your hips forward rapidly to extend your legs and toss the object upward and forward away from your body—don't throw the object straight up. If you do, get the heck out of the way! The goal is to throw it away from your body, not above your head. Ever.

Step forward with your dominant leg on the follow-through as you extend your arms. This will help simulate the motion of finishing off the tire push (i.e., stepping forward to drive it over).

Once you're throwing the object more than 8 feet away from the starting position at 4 to 6 feet above the ground, it's time for you to move up in weight.

BAND SQUAT & PRESS

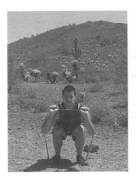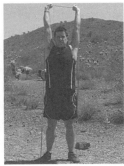

Bands are a great way to resistance train anywhere. I personally carry one or two 42-inch-long, ½-inch-thick bands with me when I travel; they're like my own portable gym! You can pick up one or a pair from nearly any fitness store or online for about $20 and get a ton of useful stretches and exercises out of them, like this one.

Place an exercise band on the ground and place the center of both feet on the band about shoulder-width apart, toes pointed slightly outward. Squat down and grab the upper loop with both hands using an overhand grip. Stretch the band by bending your elbows and raising the backs of both hands up toward your shoulders while maintaining the squatting position. Your elbows should be at your sides and your thighs should be parallel to the ground. This is the starting position.

Pushing from your heels, straighten your legs, press your hips forward, and stretch the band up by extending your arms directly overhead. Don't lock your knees or elbows.

Push your hips back slightly as if you were sitting down, bend your knees, and drop into a squat position; bend your elbows and bring them back to your side and return your hands to shoulder height, still gripping the band. That's 1 rep.

OBSTACLE TO DOMINATE
Raise the Bucket

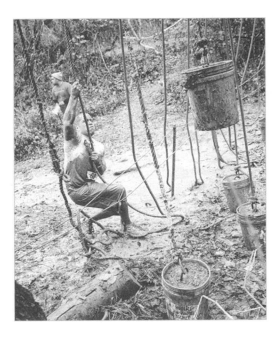

Think of this obstacle as a tug-of-war with a weight on the other end. Even using the best technique, this one will require upper-body strength and total body coordination to hoist a concrete-, water-, or stone-filled bucket 20 or more feet into the air. Like pirates raising the main sail, you'll be yanking a rope down by squatting and pulling, and there's a very good chance you'll also be shouting like a pirate, too: "AAARRRGGGHHH!"

Raise the Bucket

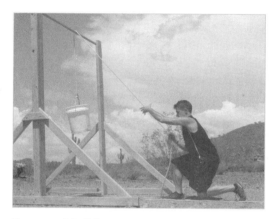

If you can't build your own apparatus to train on, perform Band Pull-Downs followed by Jumping Pull-Ups. If you can build your own, you'll be ahead of the game on race day. All you need is a bucket, some rope, and a tree branch. Make sure the branch, bucket, and rope can hold whatever weight you decide to use and you can pull the bucket up and down without dropping it on anyone or anything. Start out extremely light and work your way up; the weight of the bucket will pull you toward the object as it's being lowered, so be extremely careful as you add more weight. In addition, never, ever let go of the rope and drop the bucket—a weighted object falling on anyone's head can kill them. Safety first: Make sure there is absolutely no one in the area around the bucket. Period.

With the bucket placed on the ground and the rope over a branch, grasp the rope loosely in your hands and take 3 large steps backward, letting the rope slip through your fingers. Make sure your left foot has good traction; it'll be responsible for keeping you in position as you yank the rope down and the bucket up.

Grasp the rope tightly with both hands and step your right leg backward, dropping into a lunge position. Engage your core and pull the rope down to your waist using your upper body.

Remove one hand and reach up to grasp the rope while holding it in position with your other one. Straighten your back leg to allow you to reach higher. Dropping your hips into the lunge will help you initiate the movement each time you relocate your hands.

Repeat until the bucket is 3 feet below the tree branch—never yank the bucket to make contact with the branch—and slowly lower the bucket by using the opposite hand-under-hand movement. Keep your body in the lunge position and your core tight the entire time and fight the weight of the bucket pulling you forward. Again, don't let go of the rope and drop the bucket; only half of this workout is getting the bucket up, and the other part is lowering it down carefully. If you drop the bucket in most events, you'll have to do it over or get penalized.

SPECIFIC RAISE THE BUCKET EXERCISES

FORWARD LUNGE

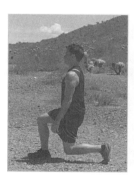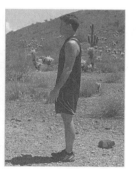

Stand tall with your feet shoulder-width apart and your arms hanging at your sides. Take a large step forward with your right foot, bend both knees, and drop your hips straight down until both knees are bent 90 degrees. Your left knee should almost be touching the ground and your left toes are on the ground behind you. Keep your core engaged and your back, neck, and hips straight at all times during this movement.

Pushing up with your right leg, straighten both knees and return to starting position.

Repeat with the other leg.

BAND PULL-DOWN

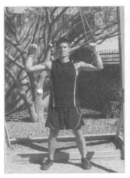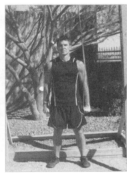

Before starting this exercise, affix the bands securely by looping them around a fixed object overhead like a pull-up bar. If you have only one band, you can perform this movement one side at a time. You can control the tension of the band for this movement by stepping forward or backward.

Grab the lower loops of the hanging bands with each hand and step backward 2 to 4 feet from the point at which the bands are attached; the bands should have enough tension to straighten out but not be fully stretched. Facing the bands' attachment points, rotate your hands so your palms face down, and close your grip around the bands. Your feet should be slightly wider than shoulder-width apart and both knees should be bent slightly so you can bend at the

waist and lean forward to place your weight on the balls of both feet. This is your starting position.

With your elbows straight but not locked, pull the bands in an arc down toward the floor and continue the motion until your arms are behind your body as far as your range of motion or the bands' tension will allow. Engage your core to prevent your body from twisting as you stretch the band in a semicircle. Hold the band in the fully stretched position for 3 to 5 seconds, then slowly return to starting position.

That's 1 rep; repeat for the indicated number of reps.

JUMPING PULL-UP

If you can perform strict-form pull-ups, good for you and go right ahead! Most folks struggle with pull-ups, and since the Strength Workout calls for Band Pull-Downs followed by Pull-Ups, being able to jump to the bar and use your momentum each time is a huge plus for most beginners or intermediate athletes. Perform Jumping Pull-Ups on a sturdy bar or playground equipment that can easily hold more than double your weight.

Align yourself under the pull-up bar, squat slightly, and jump as high as you can. Grasp the bar with either an underhand (chin-up) or overhand (pull-up) grip of your choice and use the momentum from your jump as well as the strength of your upper body to raise your chest toward the bar. Hold the bar firmly and use your core to prevent swinging as this could cause you to lose your grip and fall when you become fatigued.

If you're able to pull the bar all the way to your chest, that's optimal. Getting the bar below your chin is great, and even pulling as hard as you can after jumping and holding your body off the ground will help you build upper-body strength and get closer to performing pull-ups and even eventually muscle-ups.

OBSTACLE TO DOMINATE
Drag the Block

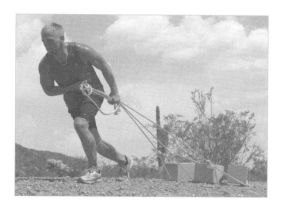

Yup, the name says it all: You're dragging a weight or a block on the end of a rope. Sometimes one, usually two, and occasionally three weighted drags through sand are on the docket, and leg strength and maintaining momentum are key to your survival.

CREATE YOUR OWN DRAGGABLE BLOCK

First off, you'll need a strong piece of rope. Make sure it's at least 6 feet long and 1/2 inch thick so you can get a good grip on it and it doesn't break on you. The easiest weight to use is an 8-inch-by-8-inch, 16-inch-long cinder block at anywhere from 24 to 35 pounds. Tie the rope securely through the holes and you're ready to start dragging. Most events will have you dragging heavy, oddly shaped objects across dirt or sand, where they'll dig in and cause friction. Do the same thing in training and don't destroy the lawn!

Some folks recommend kettlebells, but they're more expensive and because of their smooth shape are more predictable when dragging over the ground. While you do have the option to buy them in multiple weights, cinder blocks are far cheaper and closer to the real thing you'll encounter on race day.

If you choose not to create your own weight, use Weighted Backpack Sprints as an alternative to build the leg power and drive you'll need to drag the block at your next event.

MASTERING THE OBSTACLE
Drag the Block

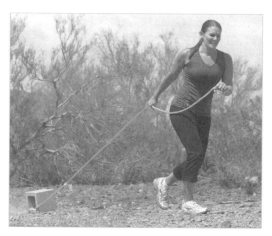

Find a dirt path or area that you can mess up pretty good by dragging around that rectangular block you fabricated. Make sure you have plenty of space to drag it in circles to complete your reps in the Strength Workout.

When first getting the block in motion, be careful not to wrench your back—that's a popular complaint for this exercise as you're usually not used to doing this in real life, aside from maybe starting up a lawn mower.

Alternate between various grips: one or two hands grasping the rope off to one side or the other, or up over the top of each shoulder. You can also turn around and walk backward holding the rope with both hands at the middle of your torso. No matter how you hold the rope or position your body, the longer you drag, the harder it'll get. The corners of the block will dig into the dirt and you'll have to dig deeply with your legs to keep the momentum moving forward and constantly tug on the rope with your arms to readjust the alignment of the block.

This exercise is not about developing some fantastic technique to make it easier to drag the block. It's about developing your strength, stamina, and confidence to be able to endure the punishment of this obstacle on race day.

SPECIFIC DRAG THE BLOCK EXERCISES

WEIGHTED BACKPACK SHUTTLE RUN

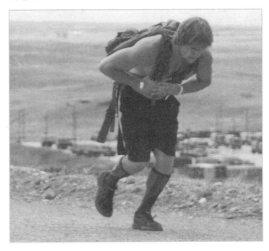

Toss some books in a backpack (in fact, I highly recommend you purchase 16 copies of this book; they make a great training tool). Whatever you put in your backpack, make sure it won't hurt your back when running. Unless you have

a super-cool backpack with a lower waist strap, it'll bounce around on your spine with each step. You may need to hold on to the straps with your hands or cross your arms over your chest to keep the backpack stable. It's supposed to be uncomfortable and difficult—you're doing this to approximate dragging a heavy block over unstable terrain!

The goal of this exercise is to develop the leg power to propel you forward as if you were dragging a block, so focus on driving forward with every step. If you want to kick it up a notch, run up a hill!

WOOD CHOP

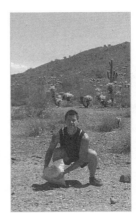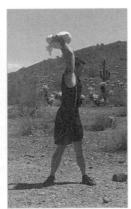

For this exercise, you can choose to use any of the weights we've covered: gallon jug, rock, log, or bucket (be careful you don't smack your face with the lip of the bucket, though!). Pick a weight that's challenging based on your athletic ability and goals. I recommend starting light while you get used to the movement.

Stand tall with your feet shoulder-width apart and hold a weight in front of you.

Lower your body into a squat until your knees are bent 90 degrees and bring the weight down to lightly touch your left foot.

Stand tall, twisting your torso to the right and lifting your arms straight up over your head. Your left shoulder should be in front and you should be looking to the right.

Repeat to the other side.

Strength Workout

	rest 2 minutes after every set (longer if required)			
Set 1	50-Yard Sandbag Carry (p. 73)	3 Tire Flips (p. 74) *or* 6 Squat & Tosses (p. 75)	16 Wood Chops (p. 80)	50-Yard Drag the Block (p. 79) *or* 100-Yard Weighted Backpack Shuttle Run (p. 80)
Set 2	50-Yard Farmer's Walk (p. 73)	20 Lunges (p. 77)	20 Band Squat & Press (p. 76)	50-Yard Farmer's Walk (p. 73)
Set 3	50-Yard Overhead Weighted Walk (p. 73)	5 Raise the Buckets (p. 76) *or* 5 Band Pull-Downs (p. 78) and 5 Jumping Pull-Ups (p. 78)	50-Yard Overhead Weighted Walk (p. 73)	5 Raise the Buckets (p. 76) *or* 5 Band Pull-Downs (p. 78) and 5 Jumping Pull-Ups (p. 78)

Dexterity Workout:
Moving Your Body Over, Under, Across, & Through Obstacles

Every obstacle that requires you to haul your ass over, under, or through it will undoubtedly require upper-body strength, coordination, and momentum employed in conjunction to get you to the other side. The great news is you can usually use a little bit more of one to make up for what you may be lacking in another.

For example, the more momentum you can employ by running up and jumping when climbing a wall, the less upper-body exertion you'll have to dole out to get up and over it. Using the right technique while climbing a rope will also help to make up for a weak grip or arm strength while still allowing you to ring the bell at the top. So the lesson for this section is to use the exercises to develop your ability and choose when to use technique, momentum, or brute force on race day.

OBSTACLE TO DOMINATE
Walls of All Shapes & Sizes

Without much hesitation, I'll confidently say that you'll encounter some of the walls in this section on race day. In most cases you'll have several to overcome! Every wall requires you to work hard get to the other side. Keeping you on one side is pretty much its entire job description. We'll cover them from easiest to hardest and give you the low-down on how to tackle walls in general and some specific tips for particular ones.

MASTERING THE OBSTACLE
Vertical Walls

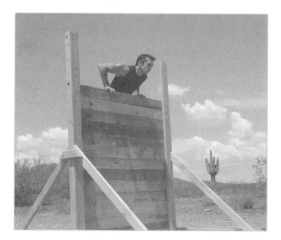

The fastest, easiest way to get over a wall is to jump straight up and grasp the top of the wall with both hands, pull down with your arms, and raise your waist up to the top of the wall, place your belly on the wall, and spin 180 degrees to swing your legs over to the other side and continue to hold the wall as you lower yourself on the back side. Now, while that sounds simple,

it requires some practice to make the movement fluid.

Placing your forearms on the face of the wall as you grip the top and raise yourself up will provide some stability. As you raise your body and bring your hands to your chest, you can place your forearms on top of the wall to give you a chance to readjust your hands or even extend one arm at a time.

Can't jump up and reach the top of the wall? Not able to pull your waist up to the top? No worry—you can use the entire obstacle to get you over the top. Many walls have a "safety step" to give you a boost so you can reach the top, and nearly every wall has braces or supports along the sides on an angle that you can grab on to. You can even grab the side of the wall itself. Is it "cheating" to use these? NO! These things are called obstacles or a reason; it's up to you to figure out how to get over them and it's smart to use all the methods that are available to you!

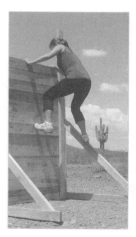 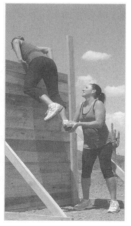

Before you attack the wall, walk up and scope out the hand/foot positions you plan on using. Approach the wall with some momentum—not a sprint, but enough speed that you can transfer your momentum upward—and place your foot securely on the safety step or the support and push off to get your hands on top of the wall. A boost from a friend is also a great way to get up! Once you have your hands firmly on the top of the wall, use your momentum to get your waist up to the top of the wall and place your belly on top. If you have to grab the side of the wall on the way up to steady yourself, go right ahead. Keeping your hands on top of the wall, spin 180 degrees, and get your feet on the opposite side of the wall. Some folks "throw" their feet over, but whatever method you use, it's important that you stay low and stable on the wall with both hands holding firmly grasping the wall. Do NOT stand up or place your feet on top of the wall; the higher your center of gravity, the less stable you are. Once you've rotated your feet to the other side, keep your hands on the wall and slowly lower yourself down to your feet by extending your arms completely before letting go of your grip.

FINDING YOUR OWN WALL FOR TRAINING

While it's not incredibly difficult to build most of the following walls, there's a good chance you can find suitable replacements. A little creativity can convert a gate or a brick wall into a training area and most parks with a playground will have structures you may be able to use. For concave walls, check out the different-size half-pipes at your local skate park to test your newly found skills.

TIP: Shoes with hard rubber toes will help you get some grip and a bit of extra leverage when climbing up vertical walls. With your hands on top of the wall, press your toes against the wall and walk them up while you pull your waist up to the top of the wall.

If you plan to build your own wall, make it modular so you can add boards to make it taller, swap a few out for a slat wall, or bolt on some studs to make a horizontal climbing wall, secure a rope up top to practice your rope climbs–you get the idea. There are step-by-step directions on www.mudrunguide.com/thewall for you to fabricate your own modular wall just like the one you see in the exercise photos. For less than $150 and a few hours of time, you can have the ultimate tool for wall climbs, pull-ups, muscle-ups, rope climbing, and more. It's up to you to convince your significant other, parents, homeowner association, or landlord that it's necessary.

MASTERING THE OBSTACLE
Angled Walls

Viewed from the side, these A-frame structures normally provide the least amount of challenge, but in cases where water or soap is added, they can prove to be a bit tricky. If it's a small wall of about 4 feet in height, you may be able to use pure momentum to carry you over it. Run toward the wall and jump off one foot enough for your opposite foot to land flat on the middle of the wall. Let the momentum carry your upper body toward the apex of the wall and place both hands on top while swinging both feet over the wall to the outside of your hands in a vaulting maneuver, or slide down the back side of the wall on your butt.

Some larger angled walls will have ropes; treat them similarly to the smaller wall above. Instead of grabbing the wall after your first step, reach down and grab the rope with both hands and quickly begin grasping hand over hand, pulling yourself up the wall while using your leg strength and momentum to run up and over it. Your momentum should be slightly forward, yet make sure your feet have good traction. On slipperier surfaces, maximize foot contact with the wall by standing nearly upright in relation to the wall and stabilizing your upper body; continue to walk your arms up the rope. This will be a little more taxing on your upper body as you'll be fighting gravity to lift more of your body weight.

Slat Walls

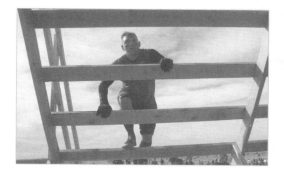

With open spaces between each wood section, these walls can be climbed not unlike a ladder—grip the slats with both hands and use the strength of your legs to climb up. Don't come at these walls with too much of a running start or you risk smashing your shins or the top of your feet on the edge of a low board; instead, take two or three steps, squat, and leap as straight up as possible and reach the highest board you can grasp firmly with both hands. Position your feet squarely on a lower board before moving your hands to the next higher slat. Maintain three points of contact with the boards at all times.

When your hands reach the top of the wall, grasp firmly and move your feet up until the wall is at waist height. Bend forward and lay your torso flat on the wall and simultaneously swing

one leg up while spinning your body 90 degrees. Use this momentum to bring your other leg over the wall as you continue to spin and maintain your grip on the top of the wall while placing your feet on a board on the opposite side of the wall. Lower yourself slowly and carefully, keeping three points of contact with the wall at all times.

Vertical Walls with Ropes

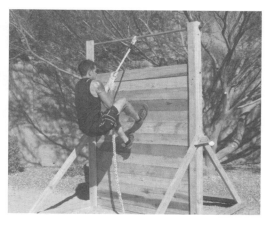

Usually the tallest walls of the bunch, vertical walls with ropes are commonly 10 to 12 feet high and feature a rope to help you scale the side of these monstrous barriers. Ropes can be knotted or not, although it's much easier if they are, and many of these obstacles will feature horizontal boards or rungs every two or three feet so you can use your legs to assist in the climb.

Use a balance of strength and technique to get you over these walls so you can conserve energy for other obstacles. To do this, you must coordinate your footing and hand-over-hand grip and pull to "walk" up the wall like the campy TV version of *Batman* from the 1960s.

When you get to the top, place both hands on the apex and pull your waist up to the top of your wall. Place your torso on the wall; spin while lifting your legs over the top (as described in "Mastering the Obstacle: Vertical Walls," page 83).

Since you're 10 or 12 feet in the air, dropping straight down would be a bad move. Keep your hands on the apex of the wall and get secure footing on a rung before you begin to lower yourself. Remember to keep three points of contact with the wall for safety.

Some obstacles have additional ropes on the opposite side of the wall to climb down. Transfer one hand at a time from the top of the wall to the rope and secure your legs or feet on the rope before descending in a controlled manner. (See "Rope Climb" on page 94 for more tips on climbing up and down ropes.)

reach and ability as a climber to help keep you on the wall till the end without falling off.

The grip of your hands will keep you on the wall as well as help you progress forward while your legs provide balance and stability to keep your forearms from doing all the work. Rest as needed, and even shake out one hand at a time if your legs are stable and your forearms are cramping up. If you're new to this type of obstacle, keep three points of contact and move your forward hand or foot first to initiate forward progress. Advanced athletes with strong grip strength may find it faster to hop both feet at the same time to a new position and then move their hands one at a time.

Move as rapidly as you can along the wall, but don't get too carried away. Some walls have loose boards or long reaches that will test your planning and execution–fools rush in (and fall).

MASTERING THE OBSTACLE
Horizontal Climbing Walls

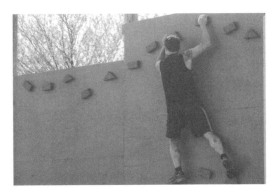

Balance and grip strength are two big factors in conquering an obstacle that can be a bit more difficult than you might expect. Plan every hand and foot position based on the length of your

MASTERING THE OBSTACLE
Concave Walls/ Half-Pipes

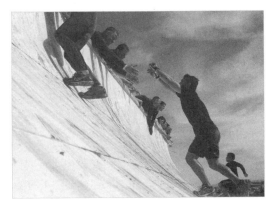

They aren't just for skaters or snowboarders anymore. These walls test your agility, leaping ability, grip, and upper-body strength like no

TIP: Learn jumping from a swimmer—no, not jumping into the water. The way a swimmer rotates his body in the water allows him to reach and pull farther above his head. If you can't jump and reach the top of the wall with both hands, twisting sideways will allow you to reach up farther with one of your hands to grab the top of an obstacle. This comes in handy as long as your single hand can grasp the top for a split second and allow you to bring your other hand up.

others. Add a slippery surface and they're quite a task to get over!

Momentum is clearly your friend in this obstacle. A running start will help you jump off one leg and plant your foot as far up the wall as possible toward the midpoint of the curve and also carry your torso toward the wall so you can reach up and grab the top. Explode as hard as you can off that planted foot in the middle of the wall straight up to the top, twist, and reach one hand as high as you can. As I described in the swimmer's tip above, twisting your torso sideways to reach with one hand will provide you with a few additional inches to grasp the top lip of the wall or a fellow competitor's hand.

Help and be helped. The code of honor in obstacle races of helping out your fellow competitors is in full effect on walls, especially concave ones. These things are downright tough for a lot of competitors who don't have a good strength-to-weight ratio to overcome. A friendly pair of hands reaching over to provide support and encouragement is a huge help. Unless you're going for the podium, help those behind you—the karma boost is completely worth it, and you may need their help on the next obstacle!

The grip your planted foot has on the middle of the wall is key to your success; if you slip there's a good chance you'll face-plant into the wall and slide down to start all over again.

Clear as much mud as possible from your shoes and pick a path that looks like it has been recently cleaned from someone sliding down (yes, you can use other's misfortunes to your benefit, so make sure you follow the tip above to pay back karma with a good deed).

If you're going it alone without a set of hands to pull you up, a strong upper body will top off the move. Hopefully, you'll still have a little bit of momentum left from pushing off your planted foot in the middle of the wall and grasp with one hand, then the other, and perform a momentum pull-up and muscle-up to get your torso flat on top of the wall. Spin around 180 degrees and secure yourself before you help others or descend the back side of the obstacle.

SPECIFIC WALL CLIMB EXERCISES

WALL CLIMB

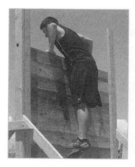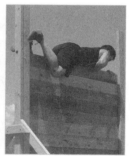

Locate any wall or structure that can support your weight safely that's approximately 6 to 8 feet in height; you should be able to grab the top and pull yourself up. You don't necessarily need to practice the "over" part—the goal of this exercise is to learn to use your momentum and develop your upper-body strength to pull your waist all the way up to the top of the wall.

Start directly in front of the wall and take 3 to 5 large steps backward, depending on how much momentum you want to put into the jump. Bound forward and jump 2 to 3 feet away from the wall, reach up, and grab the top edge with both hands. Using your momentum, pull your hands down toward your hips and extend your arms to raise your waist up to the top of the wall.

While you're up there, bend your elbows and lower your chest back down to the top of the wall before straightening your arms and pressing your waist back up to the top—it's a great way to strengthen your triceps and forearms. Repeat 3 to 5 times if you can.

Now, if you've created a wall of your own, you're lucky enough to get to practice the technique on "Mastering the Obstacle: Vertical Walls" (page 83) anytime you'd like! My favorite workout is setting a timer on my smartphone for 1:00 and counting how many times I can repeatedly get over the wall before it runs out. Take 3 steps back from the wall to start, then run, jump, climb, and descend—repeat as many times as you can. For a killer upper-body workout, take away the 3 steps and start with just a squat jump to grab the top of the wall each time.

> **TIP:** If you need a little boost, jump up slightly at the start of the move.

DOOR PULL-UP

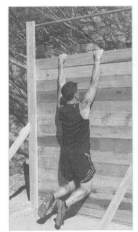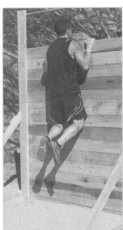

These are a great way to get some training almost anywhere and help develop the strength and skills to get over walls of all heights. I've done these in hotels everywhere I've traveled that don't have a gym, and even at some that do.

The first step is to find a door that's sturdy enough to hold at least double your weight; you'll be putting a lot of stress on it. Solid-core doors with strong hinges are a must; hollow-core doors can crack and crumble. Also make sure that the top edge isn't sharp or slippery.

Open the door in such a way to give yourself ample space to perform the exercise, and wedge a doorstop under it to keep it in place. The last thing you want to do is have the door close on your fingers!

Standing directly in front of the door, reach up and place your hands on top of the door with your forearms flat on the front of it. Using your forearms on the door as a lever, breathe out and engage the large muscles of your upper back and arms, bend your elbows, and pull your chest up to the top of the door. Inhale as you slowly lower your feet back to the ground.

Once you get the hang of it, at the top of the exercise transition one forearm and then the other flat on top of the door and extend your arms to press your waist up to the top of the door—that's only if you have space and can do so without hitting the ceiling!

LINEAR REACTIVE STEP-UP

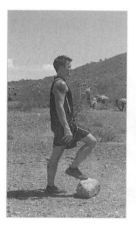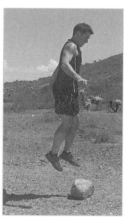

Start by standing 12 to 18 inches in front of a bench or object 18 to 24 inches tall that can hold your weight; have your hands at your sides and feet shoulder-width apart.

Step up with your right foot as if you were climbing a step and place it flat on top of the bench, leaving your left foot on the ground.

Push down with your right foot on top of the bench and jump up as high as you can using only the strength of your right leg. Your left leg should not be pushing off at all; this exercise works one leg at a time to develop explosive jumping power. Let your arms swing naturally at your sides as you jump.

Switch legs in mid-air by bringing your right foot backward and left foot forward at the apex of your jump. Your left foot will land on top of the bench and your right foot on the ground.

As soon as your left foot lands on the bench, immediately jump again using only the strength of your left leg.

That's 2 reps.

BOX JUMP

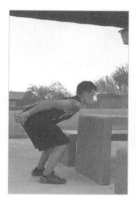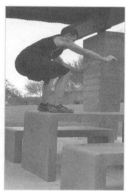

Start by standing 12 to 18 inches in front of a box or bench that's 24 to 36 inches tall and can hold your weight. Keep your hands at your sides and feet shoulder-width apart.

Initiate the jump by dropping your hips and bending at the waist in a squat movement, but only about half as deep. Swing your arms back and shift your weight toward the front of your feet.

Extend your hips, swing your arms forward, and push off from your feet to jump as high as you can toward the center top of the box. Land softly on the box with your knees bent to absorb the shock.

Step off to either side of the box, placing a hand on the edge of the box if necessary to keep your balance. Don't jump backward off the box. That's 1 rep.

BENCH DIP

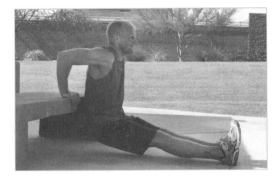

A great way to build triceps and chest strength, bench dips are also pretty convenient to do just about anywhere.

Sit on the very edge of a stable bench that can support your weight and place your palms next to your hips and grip the edge of the bench. Raise your butt off the bench and walk your feet out in front of you. Keep your legs straight and bend at your waist a little wider than 90 degrees. This is the starting position.

Inhale, bend your elbows, and slowly lower your butt down toward the floor, stopping when your upper arms are at a 90-degree angle in relation to your lower arms.

Exhale and extend your arms until they're straight, pressing your body weight up with the muscles of your upper arms. That's 1 rep.

Cargo Nets

File cargo nets under the "they look easier than they are" category of obstacles that you'll encounter on race day. These friendly looking safety nets can be spiderwebs to ensnare your arms and feet—that's what they were created for!

Cargo nets are not only great for securing heavy loads, they're essentially a "safety ladder" whereby the design will catch the arms or legs of a climber that slips and hopefully prevent a catastrophic fall. While that's reassuring, it doesn't help us get over them any more easily, but the tips below will help.

The tighter a cargo net is secured, the easier it is to climb or traverse. Unfortunately, race directors know this and usually leave them pretty loose with lots of room for you to flail your arms and legs to get up or over and really tire you out in the process.

Vertical Cargo Nets

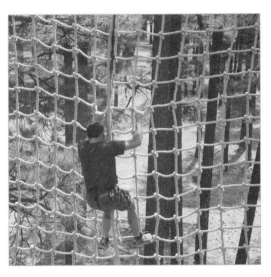

Find the seam or attachment point where the net is secured the tightest. The net will get progressively looser from there, and it's easiest to climb close to a support.

Stretch the net over a support beam, place your hands and feet on opposite sides of it, and climb like a ladder. With your weight pushing the net centered on the support beam, the net will be tight and you'll be transferring some of your weight to the beam as well—it's a win-win as far as stability and climbing speed.

If you can't find a support beam, pick a spot between other competitors—the more weight on the net, the tauter it'll be. Some extremely helpful racers may actually pull on the net to firm it up a bit, so go ahead and use it. Remember, if they help you, make sure you help them or others.

Take your time and be controlled in your movements; lift each leg clear of a cell before moving to the next one as most hang-ups are caused by missing a foot placement and falling into the net. The more you struggle, the more ensnared you'll become. If you fall into the net, count 1, 2, 3, 4—as in your hands and feet. Make sure you get each one back in position on the ropes before you try to move farther up the ladder. Dropping down a cell is always an option, especially if you don't have a lot of upper-body strength or energy to pull yourself up while trying to straighten out your foot placement.

hit other competitors or supports. Make sure the coast is clear, lower your head and shoulder, and perform a forward roll over that shoulder. Judge the speed of your roll based on how long the net is, and absolutely make sure you don't put your head into a hole in the net. Keep arms and legs tucked as much as possible to avoid snags and keep the momentum going to complete additional rolls.

If the forward roll is too fast or dangerous, a side roll is somewhat more controlled but will require more space. You're also a little more apt to catch your feet. In addition, transitioning to a forward movement from the side roll is a bit slower than from the forward roll.

If you're not able or willing to roll, a bear crawl is the best option—carefully place your hands and feet on the ropes and move one hand and the opposite leg at a time to keep your balance. Expect to be a bit frustrated with the slow progress and the number of times your hand or foot misses the rope and falls through. It may just frustrate you enough to work on your forward roll skill before the next event.

SPECIFIC CARGO NET EXERCISES

CARGO NET CLIMB

If you can locate a cargo net or even build one yourself (I've seen instructions on the Internet), you'll be able to practice to your heart's content and master this somewhat tricky obstacle that's notorious for absorbing a ton of your energy as you fight to get over it. While all cargo nets are different based on cell size and tension, developing the hand and foot coordination as well as core, arm, and leg strength in practice will absolutely help you when confronted with a cargo net on race day.

MASTERING THE OBSTACLE

Horizontal Cargo Nets

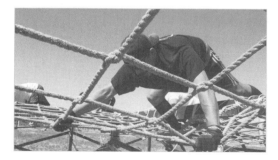

The quickest way to get across a horizontal cargo net is to tuck and roll, provided you don't

ONE-LEGGED SQUAT

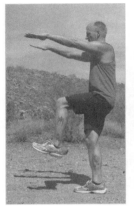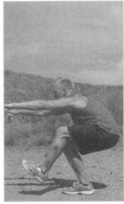

Stand with your legs slightly bent and shoulder-width apart and extend your arms in front of you for balance. Lift your left leg off the ground by bending your left knee and raising it forward at the hip. Maintain your balance directly over the middle of your right foot and begin your descent by bending at the hips and sitting back just a little bit as if you were about to sit directly down into a chair.

Next, bend your right knee slowly and keep your head up, eyes forward, and arms out in front of you for balance. As you descend, contract your glutes and continue the sitting motion while your body leans forward slightly so that your shoulders are almost in line with your right knee. Your right knee shouldn't extend past your right toes and your weight should remain between the heel and the middle of your right foot; don't roll up on the ball of your foot. Stop when your right knee is bent 90 degrees and your right thigh is parallel to the floor, and then push straight up from your right foot back to the starting position.

Don't lock your knees at the top of the exercise. Switch legs and repeat to complete 1 rep.

INCHWORM

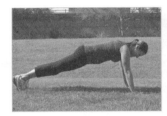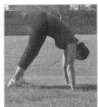

This is a great full-body exercise and a perfect test for hamstring and lower-back flexibility. In this motion-based exercise, you'll advance forward approximately 4 feet per repetition, so plan your exercise positioning accordingly.

Stand with your feet about hip-width apart and fold over so that your hands touch the floor. Keeping your hands firmly on the floor to balance your weight, walk your hands out in front of you one at a time until you're at the top of a push-up. Hold for 3 seconds.

Keeping your hands firmly on the floor to balance your weight, "walk" your feet toward your head by taking very small steps on your toes. Imagine that your lower legs are bound together and you can only bend your feet at each ankle. As you continue walking your feet toward your head, your butt will rise and your body will form an inverse "V." When you've stretched your hamstrings, glutes, and calves as far as you can, hold that position for 3 seconds.

That's 1 rep.

BICYCLE CRUNCH

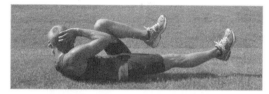

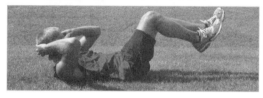

Lie flat on your back with your legs extended straight along the floor and your hands at both sides of your head, fingers touching your temples. Raise your feet 6 inches off the floor while simultaneously contracting your rectus abdominis and lifting your upper back and shoulders off the floor. In one movement, bend your left knee and raise your left leg so that the thigh and shin are at 90 degrees; rotate your torso using your oblique muscles so that your right elbow touches the inside of your left knee.

Rotate your torso back to center and lower your upper body toward the floor, stopping before your shoulders touch.

Extend your left knee and return your foot to 6 inches off the floor and bend your right leg to 90 degrees. Contract your abs, rotate, and touch your left elbow to the inside of your right knee.

That's 2 reps.

FORWARD ROLL

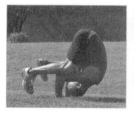

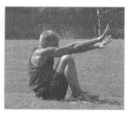

To execute the forward roll properly and efficiently, you essentially want to curl yourself up into a ball and then roll forward. While extremely helpful in quickly progressing over horizontal cargo nets, a forward roll can also come in handy if you fall forward with too much momentum when dismounting other obstacles. Simply put, it's a useful skill to learn and execute properly.

Bend your knees and squat down, lean forward slightly, and place your fingers on the floor in front of your toes. Bend your neck and bring your chin to your chest, "tucking" your head. Drop your shoulders down, rotate your pelvis forward to arch your back, and roll up onto your toes while your head is at about the level of your knees.

Push off with your toes to start the movement forward and let gravity do the rest. Keep your back arched and your head tucked until you complete the roll and your feet are back on the ground. In a cargo net, be careful not to get your hands or feet caught in the net; make sure to get your footing immediately when you complete the roll and either exit the net or complete additional rolls until you're across the obstacle.

SIDE ROLL

Also called a log roll, a side roll is something you most likely learned in grade school physical education class or at least every time you were taught to "stop, drop, and roll." Well, this is the roll part. This move is not only helpful in cargo nets but will prove invaluable in areas where you have to crawl under something (let's say barbed wire) and want to do it more quickly and less painfully than using an army crawl on your hands and knees. A side roll is a great alternative to crawling face-down in the dirt if you have enough room to turn sideways.

Start off in the top position of a push-up: hands and toes on the floor, body flat, and arms and legs extended. Initiate the move by moving your right hand across your body, using gravity to fall and roll down your right elbow and shoulder while simultaneously using your core strength and a little push-off with your left toe to twist your body and start the roll.

OBSTACLE TO DOMINATE
Rope Climb

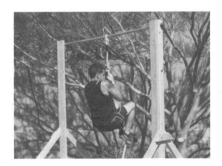

You probably hated climbing ropes in gym class back in school (I know I did!). Well, there's probably a very good reason for that: Your gym teacher was most likely teaching you the most difficult way to climb, which relied heavily on pure upper-body strength.

Also, most people think that you climb a rope by pulling up with your arms and hands. That's completely wrong—your legs and core do (or should do) most of the climbing and your hands help to keep you in place while you raise

your legs up. Essentially, you're hanging by your arms as you squat and move your feet up the rope before standing up, extending your arms, and reaching up as high as you can on the rope.

There's one exception to the above rule: If you have tremendous upper-body strength and can climb all the way to the top by just using your hands and allowing your legs to hang free, congratulations for being able to perform the fastest method for climbing a rope! You probably don't need the following info unless you're looking for a way to save some of your upper-body power for the rest of the race; arm only is fast but incredibly taxing on the arms, hands, core, and back.

For the rest of us, here are three different ways to get you up that rope. The only difference is the way you use your feet to brake or pinch the rope in order to allow you to stand up and reposition your hands higher on the rope.

MASTERING THE OBSTACLE
Rope Climb

No matter what foot position you're using, you'll be reaching up hand over hand one at a time and grasping the rope firmly. The closer you can pull your feet up toward your hands with each squat, the more vertical distance you'll cover with each movement.

Initial hand placement: Jump and extend your arms to reach and grasp the rope as high as you can with both hands, one above the other. Steady yourself on the rope while you prepare to get your feet into the position of your choice.

Foot Placement—Pinch Method: This is the best method for climbing a rope with knots; you'll pinch your feet together above the knot and "stand" on it while you reach up and reposition your hands. When climbing a rope without knots, this method is greatly dependent on the strength of your leg adductor muscles and the grip on the instep of your footwear to keep your feet locked in place on the rope. This is the most inefficient way to climb a knotless rope, resulting in wasted energy and worn-out arms, core, and legs as your feet invariably slip down the rope.

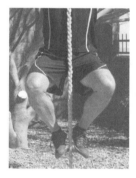

How to Do It: With your arms extended overhead and hands holding the rope tightly, squeeze both of your feet together loosely with the rope between the insteps of both feet, and bend at your waist to raise your legs as close to your hands as possible. Squeeze your feet together tightly (preferably on top of a knot) to hold your place on the rope while you extend your torso, "stand up," and reach your hands up as high as possible on the rope. Repeat until you get to the top. Use the pinching to slow your descent, lowering your hands one under the other until your feet are safely on the ground. Do not slide down the rope!

Foot Placement—Calf Wrap Method: This is commonly known as the "Marine Brake and Squat" and is much more efficient than the pinch method because the rope is held securely by wrapping it around your calf and then looping it under one and over the other foot. Famous for

rope burns, this method is best accomplished while wearing long pants or tall socks.

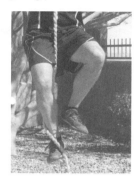

How to Do It: With your arms extended overhead and hands gripping the rope, allow the rope to hang between your legs. Rotate your right leg clockwise (counter-clockwise with your left leg if you prefer) around the rope so that it wraps around your lower leg and then the outside of your right foot. Take your left foot and loop it under the rope so that the rope is under your right foot and on top of your left. Pressing your left foot on top of your right foot to trap the rope between them acts as a brake to lock the rope in place. Release the tension between your feet and allow the rope to slide around your leg as you squat and raise your feet upward toward your hands. Clamp your left foot on top of your right to secure your foot position while you stand up and reach as high as you can to get a new grip on the rope. Repeat all the way until you reach the top of the rope. Use the foot brake to slow your descent, lowering your hands one under the other until your feet are safely on the ground. Do not slide down the rope!

Foot Placement—Tactical Speed Climb: This is undoubtedly the fastest way to climb a rope while using your feet (arm only is the fastest altogether) and has the added benefit of not resulting in as many rope burns and can be performed rather comfortably in shorts. Perfected and used by military Special Operations personnel, this method is the best choice for most obstacle racers.

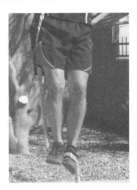

How to Do It: With your arms extended overhead and hands holding the rope, allow the rope to fall to the outside of your right leg (swap the directions for opposite legs if you prefer). Loop your left foot under the rope so that it's under your right foot and on top of your left. Press your left foot on top of your right foot and trap the rope between them to lock the rope in place. Release the tension between your feet and allow it to slide around your leg as you squat and raise your feet upward toward your hands. Clamp your left foot on top of your right to secure your foot position while you stand up and reach as high as you can to get a new grip on the rope. Repeat all the way until you reach the top of the rope. Use the foot brake to slow your descent, lowering your hands one under the other until your feet are safely on the ground. Do not slide down the rope!

SPECIFIC ROPE-CLIMBING EXERCISES

ROPE CLIMB

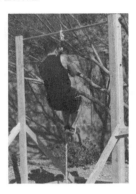

The best way to get stronger at climbing a rope is to, well, climb a rope. Using the foot placement method of your choice, practice climbing up and down to develop confidence, then strength, and finally speed. If you can't find a suitable rope, perform Towel Pull-Ups and Hanging Leg Raises to develop the upper-body and core strength needed for rope climbing. Mastering each of the different foot positions requires practice, so track down a gym in your area that has a rope or create your own. The rope I use to train was fabricated from three strands of cheap ½ inch polyester rope that I wove together to make it thick enough to grip. Secure it safely to a sturdy branch and start climbing.

TOWEL PULL-UP

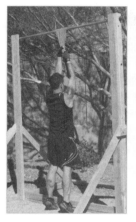
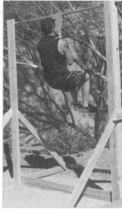

Before starting this exercise, loop a towel around a fixed overhead object like a pull-up bar. The thicker the towel is, the more difficult it'll be to grip, providing an enhanced workout for your hands and forearms. Grip the towel like a baseball bat, with both hands opposite each other.

From a hanging start, exhale and use your back and upper-body muscles to pull your hands down toward your sternum.

Pause at the top, then inhale while you lower yourself in a slow, controlled manner. Switch hands and repeat.

HANGING LEG RAISE

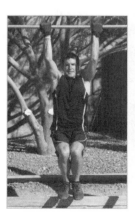
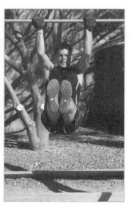

Grab an overhead bar with your preferred grip (underhand, overhand, or mixed) and hang from the bar with your arms fully extended but elbows not locked. For this exercise, count 3 seconds up, hold 1 to 3 seconds, and then count 3 seconds down.

Contracting your abdominal muscles, slowly bring your knees up toward your chest while keeping your torso as close to vertical as possible. Don't lean back during the movement or swing between reps. Slowly lower and extend your legs and hold a pike position for 3–5 seconds with each rep.

Lower your legs in a slow and controlled manner. That's 1 rep.

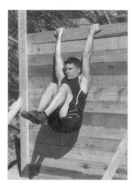

Variation: If you don't have a bar, you can use a sturdy door or equivalent. Place your back against the door, reach up, and grasp the top of the door with a supinated overhand grip.

OBSTACLE TO DOMINATE
Mud Pits & Muddy Slopes

In some events, this is the whole reason you signed up: to get muddy! In others, it's just that extra little bit of misery to deal with between other more sinister-looking man-made contraptions. It's exactly because of this that mud pits don't necessarily get their due as a difficult obstacle unto themselves—that is, until you're up to your neck in it!

Mud Pits & Muddy Slopes

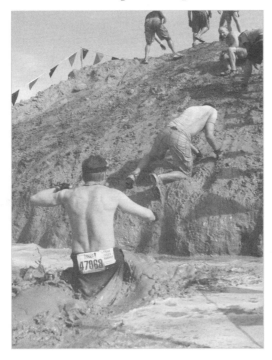

Finish-line mud pits are usually the deepest, thickest goop on the course. Of course, this isn't a universal rule, but most races save the big splash for last so that fans can cheer and you can make a jackass out of yourself. Also, your face full of mud makes the celebratory beer taste even better.

How do you get through it? You get down on your elbows and knees and army crawl. You may need to use your hands or even stand to keep your head above the brown soup, but there's no real trick or skill to the mud pit—just get through it as quickly as you can by keeping your momentum the entire time. If you can use some momentum from running up to the pit and taking an extremely shallow, head-first, hands-extended slide (note: never, ever dive) as if you were doing a Pete Rose impersonation stealing second base, that'll help you slide even farther. If there's barbed wire strung over the top of the pit, make sure to keep your head, butt, and limbs down until you're completely clear of it!

The finish-line mud pit gets all the glory, with fans cheering you on and begging for a belly flop. (Don't do it. Seriously, they're laughing *at you*, not *with you*!) The end in sight also causes an endorphin rush and sears that final romp in the muck into your memory. However, the "in and out" mud pits with muddy slopes are dastardly little devils that usually prove to be one of the most difficult an d energy-sucking obstacles of each race. What are they? Dirt pile, mud pit, dirt pile, mud pit, over and over! If the injustice of getting soaking wet and muddy isn't enough, the climb out of the pit is sometimes steep and always slippery; if you lose your grip or footing, you'll slide right back down into the muck. In order to get up the other side, use your momentum, a powerful jump to start your climb, and some careful planning when choosing a route. It also never hurts to have a buddy push you out of the pit or pull you up by your arm from the other side.

Choosing your route is key. Your goal is to get through as quickly as possible, so you'll want a path that's free of slower competitors and has ample places to pull yourself up with your hands and to place your feet to finish off the climb. Quickly scan the pit to see where other competitors have successfully climbed out and if you can tell the depth of a certain area based on how deep it is on an average person's body. Most pits of this nature are dug with a backhoe, so there's a good chance the sides of the pit may not be as deep as the middle. Another reason to avoid the middle: that's where most racers before you have run through and deepened the pit as well as worn down and made the center of the next hill even more slippery. Often the sides are the quickest paths.

Use your momentum by descending the down-slope before you enter the mud pit and jump as far as you possibly can toward the far end of the pit. The less time you have to spend wading through the muck, the faster you'll be. As soon as your feet hit the bottom, if you're close enough, squat and jump as high as you can up the wall of the next dirt mound. If not, raising your feet as high as you can will provide less resistance as you continue to step forward toward the next climb.

When ascending a muddy slope, grip is obviously vital and the first foothold is the most important mooring for you to establish. Locate a suitable place for your foot to grip and jump as high as you can while reaching and clawing at the mud with your hands while you attempt to get one foot into place. It won't be easy and you may fail and slide backward, but persistence (and a push or pull from a fellow racer) pays off. Always remember the code: Help others and it'll most certainly come back to you elsewhere in the race!

SPECIFIC MUD PIT EXERCISES

ARMY CRAWL

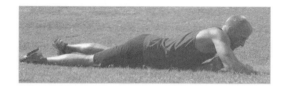

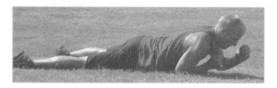

Begin flat on your stomach with your legs extended behind you and your palms and forearms on the ground at shoulder height; your elbows are bent a little more than 90 degrees. The goal is to walk forward on your forearms and knees or toes while limiting the drag of your torso on the ground. Rotate your shoulder to raise your left arm just past your head while bending your right knee, rotating your right hip, and raising your right knee up toward your right elbow.

Press your left forearm and hand into the ground to raise your torso while rotating your opposite hand and leg into position, continually moving forward.

BEAR CRAWL

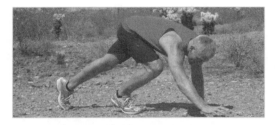

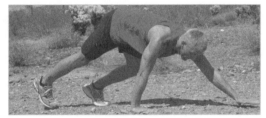

Although your butt's higher off the ground than using an Army Crawl, the Bear Crawl is effective to rapidly move under waist-high objects and is a pretty darn good full-body and core workout.

Start on your hands and knees, lift your hips up to place your toes on the ground, and extend your right arm to reach forward with your right hand and place it on the ground; simultaneously bend your left knee and rotate your left hip to bring your left knee close to your left elbow. Repeat with the opposite arm and hand to continue to move forward.

AIR SQUAT

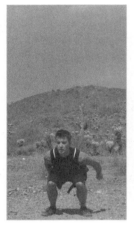 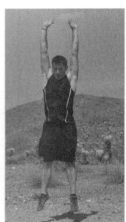

These are exactly as the name implies—squats where you catch some air. Stand tall with your feet shoulder-width apart and toes pointed slightly outward, about 11 and 1 o'clock. Raise your arms until they're parallel to the floor.

Bend at the hips and knees and sit back just a little bit as if you were about to sit directly down into a chair. Keep your head up, eyes forward, and arms out in front of you for balance. As you descend, contract your glutes while your body leans forward slightly so that your shoulders are almost in line with your knees. Your knees should not extend past your toes and your weight should remain between the heel and the middle of your feet—do not roll up on the balls of your feet during this portion of the exercise. Stop when your knees are at 90 degrees and your thighs are parallel to the floor. Swing your arms down so both hands are behind your body. Rapidly bring your arms forward in an arc and up over your head as you transfer your weight to your forefeet and explosively jump straight up in the air.

Land softly on your feet, bending your knees to absorb the impact. That's 1 rep.

Dexterity Workout

Do as many reps as possible in the time given;
rest 2 minutes after every set (longer if required)

Set 1	1:00 Wall Climb (p. 87) *or* 1:00 Door Pull-Ups (p. 88)	25-Yard Army Crawl (p. 99)	10 Inchworms (p. 92)	25-Yard Bear Crawl (p. 100)
Set 2	2:00 Cargo Net Climb (Up, Down, Left, & Right) (p. 91) *or* 5 One-Legged Squats each side (p. 92) & Jumping Pull-Up/Hang (p. 78)	22 Bicycle Crunches (p. 93)	3 Forward Rolls (p. 93)	10 Box Jumps (p. 89)
Set 3	1:00 Rope Climb (p. 94) *or* 12 Band Pull-Downs (p. 78) & 14 Hanging Leg Raises (p. 97)	15 Bench Dips (p. 90)	5 Side Rolls (p. 93)	16 Linear Reactive Step-Ups (p. 89)

Speed & Endurance Workout:
Explosive Speed, Power, & Endurance to Torch the Course

They're called "mud runs" for a reason, right? I've yet to see an event with escalators or conveyer belts to transport you from one obstacle to the next, so prepare to do some running or jogging when you sign up for a mud run or obstacle race. In fact, all of these events measure their courses in distance—from 5K to as much as 26.2 miles—and you'll need to cover all that ground as quickly as you can before tackling each and every obstacle standing in your way. This workout is designed to develop your speed through progressively more difficult sprint intervals, increase your endurance with tempo and medium-paced runs, and build your overall strength with a total-core regimen and running-specific drills.

OBSTACLE TO DOMINATE
Off-Road Running

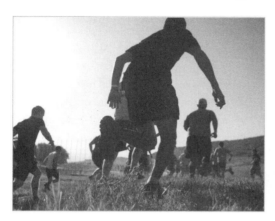

Trail running is much more challenging than a simple jog on the road—every footfall will result in uneven terrain with rocks or ruts while the elevation can change significantly from one stride to the next. Your hips, ankles, and core get more work than they ever would on a sidewalk, and every supporting muscle you never considered is forced to carry some of the load to keep you on your feet while sprinting across the undulating landscape.

The concept of pacing flies out the window and you're forced to monitor your power output by perceived exertion. This ain't your average trot in the park and needs to be treated as a completely different form of running altogether. Trail running isn't necessarily about putting in mileage—it's about putting in hard work.

MASTERING THE OBSTACLE
Off-Road Running

The first step (pun intended) is to find suitable terrain to train. It can be an off-road jogging path, a fire road, or even a jagged mountain trail. Try to find the same type of conditions that you'll face on race day to prepare properly.

Once you've picked your spot, make sure you take it easy on your first run. On harder trails, expect to run as much as 50% slower than your normal on-road pace. If you're used to running an 8-minute mile, be prepared to run at 12 minutes per mile.

There's a technical aspect to trail running: You'll take smaller, quicker strides than you would on the road and are forced pay attention to where your feet land and what they're landing on. It's extremely easy to roll an ankle on the side of a rock or trip over a root and land on your face when on the trail. If you've ever tripped on a sidewalk, then be doubly careful when trail running. Look at the trail 6 to 12 feet in front of you; don't stare at your feet.

Keep your arms away from your body to maintain your balance on rough terrain. On loose dirt or gravel, the lower your arms and hands are, the lower your center of gravity will be. Practice using light, quick steps when traversing rocky or uneven terrain; move your feet quickly across the difficult stuff to keep your balance.

Stay under control when descending a hill. The more momentum you have, the harder you hit the ground if you get out of control! Once you're at a comfortable speed, harness that momentum to get up and over the terrain in front of you.

Although they'll tire quickly at first, your ankles, knees, and back will become stronger the more time you spend off-road. Couple your trail running with some of the drills in the Speed & Endurance Workout and you'll also become a faster and more efficient runner, too.

Running in Water

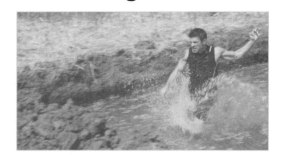

Here's what I remembered from my ninth-grade science class: Water is approximately 800 times denser than air, so running through water is an absolute boatload more difficult than normal running. While I'm not sure that "boatload" is the correct terminology, let's agree that running from point A to point B in water will be slower, harder, and drain a lot more energy than covering that distance on flat ground.

Running in Water

The key to moving as efficiently as possible is to minimize drag as much as possible—the more streamlined your body and clothes are in the water, the less resistance and effort you'll have to use to keep progressing. Tight-fitting, pocket-less shorts or pants are optimal for creating less turbulence and drag in the water, as are small, lightweight shoes with a slick surface. This is one obstacle where the Borat man-thong costume comes in especially handy; the closer you look to a swimmer, the better.

To reduce drag in water that's less than thigh deep, lift one leg completely out of the water with each step and plant it as far forward as you can, being careful not to step on submerged rocks or branches. Falling on your face will really slow you down! It'll take a little practice to get your balance, but clearing one leg and foot will cut your drag in half and allow you to get across the water more quickly. Yes, it'll use more energy, so you need to decide whether you're going for speed or feel like taking a wade through the muck.

Swimming is always an option if the water is free from debris and at least waist deep. Doggy paddle is most likely the safest option as you can keep your head out of the water to watch for other competitors, rocks, branches, and such as well as place your hands and toes on the bottom to keep you moving forward. Think of this move as a Bear Crawl in water—use your torso's buoyancy to float while you push off the bottom or paddle your hands forward.

Running from Zombies

Your brains are safe, but your pride isn't. In Run For Your Lives, if the zombies pursuing you on the course rip all three of your flags off your belt, you effectively "lose" and are zombie meat. I'm sure you didn't sign up, prepare, and show up on race day to walk away a loser, right? Well, it's time you break out some long-forgotten skills from old playground games like dodge ball, flag football, or tag that you played as a kid.

MASTERING THE OBSTACLE

Running from Zombies

Lateral movements combined with balance and flexibility are the best way to dodge, duck, dip, dive, and…er, dodge a zombie on the course. The "20/20" Drill below will have you performing plyometric moves in forward, backward, and side-to-side planes to strengthen your legs and hips while also helping you build your speed and endurance.

SPECIFIC RUNNING EXERCISES

20/20 DRILL

Speed, strength, flexibility, and endurance–these all add up to enhanced athletic performance and the ability to torch any course you set foot on. The 20/20 Drill will combine eight moves at high intensity to develop your skills and help get you in the best shape of your life.

The set-up is simple: Find a flat(ish) field at least 20 yards long and place some cones or markers at each end. Perform each of the following movements back to back with little or no rest in between. Run 20 yards out, turn around, and run 20 yards back—simple. The hard part is finding your rhythm and pushing yourself to keep the intensity up for of each of these 8 movements.

"I joked afterwards to my friends after I'd completed my first obstacle race that 'I hit a wall,' and they asked, 'At what mile?' I said, 'No, I hit a wall. It was about 9 feet tall.' I'll never forget how it felt to land on the other side and just keep going."
—Carrie Adams, founder, Rad Racing

HIGH KNEES

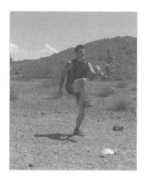

Run forward using a normal-length stride. Bend the knee of your elevated leg 90 degrees and raise it until it's level with your waist. Push forward from the ball of your grounded foot, switch legs, and repeat. Pump your arms to generate leg drive and speed.

When you've completed 20 yards of High Knees, turn around and perform Butt Kicks back to the starting position.

BUTT KICKS

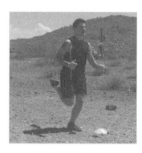

Run forward by taking very small steps and raising the heel of your back leg up toward your buttocks. Push forward from the ball of your grounded foot, progressing 12 to 18 inches per stride.

Turn around and perform 20 yards of Striders.

STRIDERS

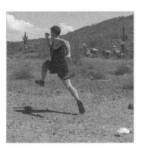

Bound forward by pushing off hard from the ball of your grounded foot, pumping your arms to generate leg drive and speed. Take huge leaps forward, trying to cover as much ground as possible with each stride.

After you've finished 20 yards of Striders, turn around and Skip back to the starting position.

SKIP

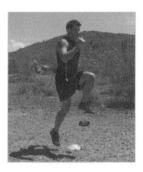

Bound forward by pushing off hard from the ball of your grounded foot, landing again on that same foot, and pushing off once more before landing on the opposite foot. Pump your arms to generate leg drive and speed. Take smaller leaps forward than when performing Striders, covering slightly less ground per stride.

Turn sideways and perform 20 yards of Side Shuffle.

SIDE SHUFFLE

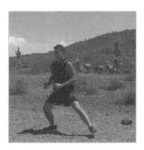

Turn sideways with your left hip pointing toward the direction you'll be traveling, feet slightly wider than your shoulders and hands at your sides. Push off with your right foot in the direction you'll be traveling while lifting your left foot and swinging your right foot toward the center of your body. Touch both feet together lightly before landing on your right foot, extending your left foot out to the side in the direction you're traveling and repeating the process.

When you reach the 10-yard mark, turn 180 degrees so that your right hip is pointing in the direction that you're traveling and continue side shuffling an additional 10 yards.

Once you've completed 20 yards, turn to face the starting position and perform 20 yards of Walking Lunges.

WALKING LUNGE

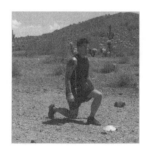

Stand tall, facing the direction you'll be traveling, with your feet shoulder-width apart and your arms hanging at your sides. Take a large step forward with your right foot, bend both knees, and drop your hips straight down until both knees are bent 90 degrees. Your left knee should almost be touching the ground and your left toes are on the ground behind you. Keep your core engaged and your back, neck, and hips straight at all times during this movement.

Keeping your right foot in place on the ground, push up with your right leg, straighten both knees, bring your left leg parallel with your right, and place your left foot next to your right.

Continue moving forward by repeating the above process with your left foot.

When you reach the start line, continue facing the same direction as you did during the Walking Lunge and perform Backward Sprints for 20 yards.

BACKWARD SPRINT

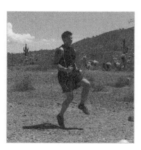

Facing away from the direction you'll traveling, run by pushing off alternating forefeet and raising your knees as high as possible. Pump your arms as needed to generate leg drive and speed. This takes a little getting used to but it's a great way to strengthen your running muscles by working them in an opposite plane of motion and helps to develop balance and agility.

Once you've reached the 20-yard mark, lower your hand to the ground with both knees bent in a starter's stance and then sprint as hard as you can back to the starting line.

SPRINT

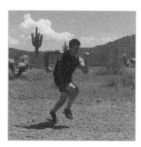

The sprint is saved for last so you're working extremely hard to generate speed after your legs and lungs are already fatigued. Run forward at top speed by leaning forward with your upper body to as much as a 45-degree angle and driving off the balls of your feet as hard and as rapidly as you can. Pump your arms to increase leg drive and speed.

RUN INTERVALS

These intervals will help you build up your mileage with two tempo runs of 1 mile each as well as 10 minutes of jogging to warm up and cool down. The hard sprints will help you develop speed and strength. When combined with the walking intervals, they'll help you get used to "switching gears" during an obstacle race or mud run when you need to get past other runners or get over, around, or through an obstacle quickly.

Jog 5 minutes at an easy pace to warm up; rest for 1:00, hydrate, and stretch your hips, calves, and quads.

Run 1 mile at a moderate pace; rest for 1:00.

Run :40 at a hard pace, walk for :30.

Run :30 at a hard pace, walk for :30.

Run :20 at a hard pace, walk for :30.

Run :10 at a hard pace, rest for 1:00.

Run 1 mile at a moderate pace.

Jog 5 minutes to cool down.

If this exercise seems too easy and the durations aren't long enough, you aren't putting enough effort into the "hard" runs.

RELATIVE PACE DESCRIPTIONS

Easy: You should be able to carry on a conversation and breathe relatively normally. An easy pace is good for warm-up, cool-down, recovery the day or two after a hard-run race, or when running long distances. Easy runs or jogs are roughly 50% of your maximal effort.

Moderate: Your breathing should be faster than normal due to your elevated heart rate and exertion. While you can't carry on a full conversation, you can speak in occasional sentences. Moderate, or tempo, runs help to build strength and endurance. Moderate runs are about 70 to 80% of your maximal effort.

Hard: This is all-out sprinting. You'll be breathing extremely hard and unable to speak more than a word or so at a time. Hard intervals are done for a short period of time to build speed and train fast-twitch muscle fibers to respond even when fatigued. Hard runs represent 95% of your maximal effort.

Speed & Endurance Workout

	rest 2 minutes after every set (longer if required)			
Set 1	20/20 Drill (p. 105)	--	--	--
Set 2	20 Hip Raises (p. 134)	14 Supermans (p. 136)	12 Bird Dogs (p. 136)	22 Marching Twists (p. 133)
Set 3	Run Intervals (p. 107)	--	--	--

Mental Preparation:
What the Hell Are You Thinking?

Friday afternoon before your first/biggest/hardest race, you'll most likely let a few co-workers or friends know what your plans are for the weekend. That is, assuming you haven't been blathering about it for the last few weeks to anyone who'll reluctantly lend you their ear.

It's all good. You need the positive and negative energy from all the well-wishers and boo-birds. Take it all in. Let the well-wishers be your safety net, you know you have supporters in your court. Use those naysayers who say "You're nuts!" as motivation that you have something to prove—not to them, but to yourself. That last bit is important: You're doing this for yourself first, and secondly to make others proud, raise money for charity, or even as a tribute to a fallen Spartan. You're the one that needs to show up and compete—make sure to prepare your mind and body and toe the line with the right training and can-do attitude.

"You Can Doooo Iiiiiit!"

Nearly every Adam Sandler movie that I can think of has a requisite cameo from Rob Schneider imploring the protagonist, usually Sandler himself, with the simple one-liner: "You can dooooo iiiiit!" Well, you can. Channel your inner voice. Repeat that simple phrase to drive you when you wake up on race morning, during the long trek from the parking lot to the check-in, as you take your place in the starting corral, and under, over, across, and through every bit of that course. Crush doubt the second it creeps into your conscious mind with that simple mantra. Destroy fear by unleashing your desire, passion, and drive to deliver on the promise you made to yourself when you clicked that hyperlink to register. Repeat it three, five, or six hundred times if you need to continually remind yourself; write it on your forearm with permanent marker if you think you might forget it! Got your own phrase? Go with that instead, as long as it'll motivate you to work your ass off and not hesitate for one second and let your commitment fade. Also, keep it short; your brain will be a little busy and the simpler, the better. Extra points if you tattoo your power phrase somewhere on your fleshy real estate; I have my own little ritual of writing "Tenacious" on my left forearm with a permanent marker before races. That's my mindset as I power through the highs and lows of endurance events toward the finish line.

Endorphin Roller Coaster: The Highs & Lows

Have you heard of "hitting the wall" in a marathon somewhere around the 20-mile mark? While that "wall" may be a physical limitation for some, for the most part it is entirely mental. In any type of endurance event, your mind can be your best friend and your worst enemy—all in the span of a few minutes. There'll be amazing highs when you conquer a difficult obstacle or pass other competitors, followed immediately by the lows—fear, doubt, outright anger toward other competitors, the course, or that rock in your right shoe that's driving you insane. The worst part? You'll have no advance warning when that dark wave will come crashing down upon you. Even during the best race of your life, as you push your body, your mind will fluctuate between light and dark. These highs and lows are relatively universal in endurance racing, so you're not going nuts if you alternate between Dr. Jekyll and Mr. Hyde out on the course.

The best way to deal with these waves is to enjoy the highs while being careful not to push yourself too hard while you're feeling like a superhero. Maintain your pace and keep your excitement under control so you don't waste valuable energy that you'll need for the rest of the race. When the lows come, you need to breathe deeply, relax, and remind your neurons who's in charge. If the thought of quitting pops into your head, just remember how far you've come and how bummed you'll be later if you bow out now.

OBSTACLES = OPPORTUNITIES

You chose this race for a reason, whether it was to conquer the mayhem with your friends, set a new personal level of excellence, or just to impress that high school heartthrob that you just friended on Facebook. There's also a pretty good chance you've obsessed over the course map and obstacle list on their website since you made that pivotal decision and are either relishing or dreading certain obstacles. Now's the best time to prepare your mind and body to get you over, under, across, and through them all. The last section gave you the mantra or power thought, and you need to couple that with the commitment to attack each barrier in order to conquer it. By commitment, I mean jumping, pulling, pushing, dragging, and running with the certainty that you have the strength, drive, and ability to crush anything that stands in your way. You need to commit to succeed; you can't dangle your toe in the water—you need to focus on trusting in yourself and your abilities and jump in with both feet. Every single obstacle gives you the opportunity to prove you're up to the challenge and build your confidence, so "leave it all on the course" by giving every obstacle your best effort devoid of the caustic limiters of your ability: fear and trepidation. Crush it.

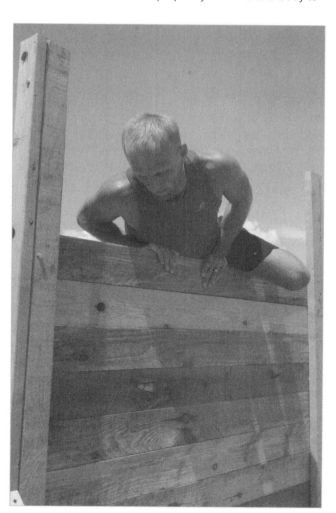

Getting Your Body Ready to Compete

If this is the first time you're hearing the term "functional cross-training," welcome to the world of calisthenics. Yes, your middle-school gym teacher wasn't nuts when she told you that true strength did require weights. Pushing and pulling your own weight is all you need to build total-body fitness and the strength to conquer any sport and truly build an impressive physique. Bulging muscles are great for show and wonderful for lifting heavy weights, but functional cross-training, or FXT, puts every muscle in your body under tension through a wide range of motion.

From the dozens of muscles that are used just to get you out of bed in the morning to that little leap/stretch maneuver to stick your hand in front of the elevator sensor to keep the doors from closing, multi-plane, full-range-of-motion exercises prepare you for real life. Try pulling and clicking your seat belt without activating your core and upper-body muscles. You can't. FXT is and always will be part of your life. Now you know it.

How do you incorporate functional cross-training into your workouts? It's very simple: Put down the weights (well, some of them) and use the most amazing functional workout machine ever invented—your body. Lucky for you, it's always conveniently located wherever you are. The Strength, Dexterity, and Speed & Endurance workouts are all functional cross-training and, simply put, you can do them nearly anywhere, anytime. Go ahead, you have my permission to knock out a set of push-ups and squats at your desk and a few chin-ups on the monkey bars at the park. I'm proud to be the impetus for the occasional strange glance you may get and happy to be the brunt of your excuse: "Brett told me to!"

> **TIP:** If you feel you're able to complete a 5K-distance event then go ahead. The programs and obstacle descriptions will make even more sense after you've already been out on the course and faced some of them yourself!

Crush the Most Bad-Ass Courses

Hopefully by now your competitive fires are stoked and you want to get out and tackle any one of the adventures outlined in the book. So, where do you start? Back in "Before You Sign Up" (page 20), we covered the necessity of preparing your body for the challenges you'll encounter at any obstacle race or mud run. Each race will present its own series of barriers and roadblocks for you to conquer, and we've designed a training plan to get you in race shape. First-timers should follow the 2-week Prep Program (page 116) and begin to build up the strength, agility, and endurance it takes to tackle the 3-week regimen of Domination Level Alpha. The advanced 5-week CRUSH IT Program is exactly what you'd expect: a full-body exercise program to kick your ass into gear for competing on the highest level—from dominating your age group to getting some hardware on the podium.

Ready? Let's get started!

Initial Test: Check Your Level of Awesomeness

This will be a timed test. Any watch or timer will do. Seconds aren't important—yet. You can perform this test outside or using a treadmill; you'll be covering up to 3 total miles, so plan your route accordingly. Start the initial test with a 3- to 5-minute warm-up using some of the moves on page 142.

INITIAL TEST EXERCISES

PUSH-UP

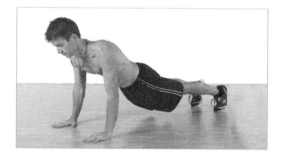

Place your hands on the ground approximately shoulder-width apart, making sure your fingers point straight ahead and your arms are straight but your elbows aren't locked. Step your feet back until your body forms a straight line from head to feet. Your feet should be about 6 inches apart with the weight in the balls of your feet.

Engage your core to keep your spine from sagging; don't sink into your shoulders.

Inhale as you lower your torso to the ground and focus on keeping your elbows as close to your sides as possible, stopping when your elbows are at a 90-degree angle or your chest is 1 to 2 inches from the floor.

Using your shoulders, chest, and triceps, exhale and push your torso back up to starting position.

SQUAT

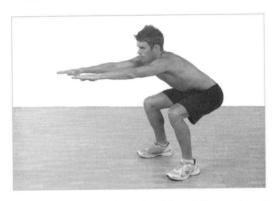

Stand tall with your feet shoulder-width apart and toes pointed slightly outward, about 11 and 1 o'clock. Raise your arms until they're parallel to the floor.

Bend at the hips and knees and "sit back" just a little bit as if you were about to sit directly down into a chair. Keep your head up, eyes forward, and arms out in front of you for balance. As you descend, contract your glutes while your body leans forward slightly so that your shoulders are almost in line with your knees. Your knees should not extend past your toes and your weight should remain between the heel and the middle of your feet—do not roll up on the balls of your feet. Stop when your knees are at 90 degrees and your thighs are parallel to the floor. If you feel your weight is on your toes or

heels then adjust your posture and balance until your weight is in the middle of your feet.

Push straight up from your heels back to starting position. Don't lock your knees at the top of the exercise. This is 1 rep.

Round 1: Start your timer—it'll run for the duration of all three rounds, including any rest breaks you may take. Rest if needed, and make sure you have water to stay hydrated.

- 5 Push-Ups
- 5 Squats
- Run, jog, or walk 1 mile at a "conversational" pace, one at which you could chat a bit with a friend, one to two sentences at a time. On a perceived exertion scale, this should be about a 5.

Optimal time for completion of Round 1 is under 15:00.

Move as quickly as you can from round to round. Take a sip of water and catch your breath, but don't forget that you're on the clock.

Round 2:

- 5 Push-Ups
- 5 Squats
- Run, jog, or walk 1 mile at a moderate pace. This isn't an all-out effort, but you shouldn't be talking more than 5 to 6 words at a time while running or walking briskly. On a perceived exertion scale, this should be about a 7.

Optimal time for completion of Round 1 is under 13:00.

Move as quickly as you can from round to round. Take a sip of water and catch your breath. The clock is still ticking!

Round 3:

- 5 Push-Ups
- 5 Squats

- Run, jog, or walk 1 mile at an overall moderate pace, adding in 2 to 3 sections where you pick up the pace. These sections can be as long as 1 minute each or as short as "until that next mailbox" while outside of "during this entire commercial" on the treadmill with a TV handy. The intensity of this pick-up interval should be an 8, not a full-out sprint (Day 1 and you're already doing interval training—yay, you!).

Optimal time for completion of Round 1 is under 12:00.

Stop your timer, that's it! Grab a towel and wipe off while drinking some water or a mixture of 50% water, 50% sports drink if you're a heavy sweater in hot conditions. Forty minutes is right around the time you should be replacing some electrolytes and a bit of glucose, but you shouldn't need a full bottle of high-calorie sports drink.

How'd you do?

Less than 30 minutes: You're a Rock Star! Start with the 5-week CRUSH IT Program on page 122. You can even jump right into the second week if you'd like! If you haven't already done a race, you're a good candidate for your first one very soon—24 days will provide you enough time to work through the final three weeks of CRUSH IT, rest for a few days, and go tackle the course of your choosing!

Less than 35 minutes: Awesome job, you're ready to start with the 5-week CRUSH IT Program on page 122. Depending on your confidence, you can sign up for an event that's around 38 days away, giving you time to complete CRUSH IT and give your body some rest or even tackle a 5K Mud Run in the next few weekends to get one under your belt.

Less than 40 minutes: Great work! You hit the optimal target for each round, and are ready for Domination Level Alpha. Follow the DLA plan and you'll be ready for a short-distance 5K Mud Run event in about 24 days. This will give you enough time to complete the 3-week program and allow your body to rest and recover for a few days before you kick it into gear.

Over 40 minutes: You just totally destroyed every single person plopped on the couch; give yourself some credit for an awesome job. All those other fast folks below 40 have stopped reading now, so let me share a secret: You're right in my wheelhouse and my favorite athletes to train—no lie! I've worked with elite athletes and professional triathletes, and I can tell you hands-down that individuals in this bracket have the most to gain and make the biggest strides over the course of any program. Welcome to my team, I'm happy you're on board. I've created a simple Prep Program on page 116 for you to follow and get you ready for Domination Level Alpha.

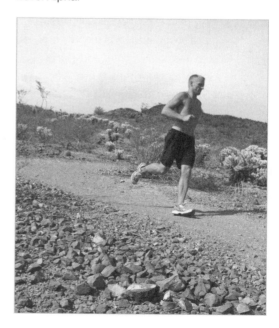

Prep Program

Welcome to the starting blocks. You're in the race from the couch to your first event and we're going to get you there faster than you ever thought possible. Congratulations on taking the first step toward a healthier future and get ready for some real excitement, some sore muscles, and the opportunity to transform your body!

Jogging and walking is going to become a big part of your regimen. As I covered on page 102, they're called mud runs for a reason. These events are based around locomotion of the human variety—you need to haul yourself from one obstacle to the next as fast as you can. Of course, "fast" is a relative term and the goal here is to help you find your optimum pace. Whether it takes three weeks or 6 months, if you stick with the program you'll continue to make progress and get that much closer to your goals of race-day domination.

This 2-week program is progressive and relative to your athletic ability; you set your own pace and ratchet up the intensity at your own speed. At the end of week two, you'll perform the Initial Test all over again and record your time—40:00 or less on the timer and you're absolutely ready for Domination Level Alpha; above that time you can repeat this program as often as you need to get ready for the DLA challenge. Even if you don't break 40 minutes after two, three, or four 2-week sessions of the Prep Program, you can decide when you're ready to move on to Domination Level Alpha.

Perform this program three times a week with at least one rest day in between. Jog at a pace that's comfortable and your heart rate and breathing is slightly elevated. Slow down if you're fatigued; stop altogether if you feel dizzy, lightheaded, or short of breath. Only resume if your breathing has returned to normal and call it a day and rest as long as you need to in order to feel OK enough to hit the showers. Don't stress out; this is like batting practice—even professional ballplayers will foul off the easy pitches quite a bit and rarely hit a home run on the first swing.

Start each training session with a three- to 5-minute warm-up, choosing some moves from the descriptions starting on page 142, and end the workout with at least 5 minutes of stretching.

TESTING YOUR PROGRESS

Retake the Initial Test (page 113) and record your time. As I mentioned earlier, 40:00 or less is optimal, but the most important aspect is for you to be delivering your best and to ensure you're ready for the challenges of Domination Level Alpha. If you're confident in your performance on the test and have completed the Prep Program a couple of times, make the call if it's time for you to move on to DLA or repeat the Prep Program following the Progression below.

REPEATING THE PREP PROGRAM–PROGRESSION

When starting the Prep Program over after taking the Week 2 Test, take at least one full day of rest and begin at Day 1 again. This time you'll be adding :10 to the duration of every walk and jog segment and 1 to 2 reps of the functional cross-training exercises. Each time you repeat the Prep Program, add this additional time and exercise reps.

Prep Program *week 1*

Note: Rest and recovery are vital to the success of the program and should be included as prescribed on the schedule.

MON	TUE	WED	THU	FRI	SAT	SUN
1:00 Walk		1:00 Walk		:35 Jog		:40 Jog
:30 Jog		:35 Jog		:45 Walk		:40 Walk
1:00 Walk		:45 Walk		:35 Jog		:40 Jog
:30 Jog		:35 Jog		:45 Walk		:40 Walk
1:00 Walk		:45 Walk		:35 Jog		:40 Jog
rest 1:00		:30 Jog		:45 Walk		:40 Walk
10 Hip Raises (p. 134)		1:00 Walk		12 Hip Raises (p. 134)		12 Bird Dogs (p. 136)
5 Squats (p. 114)		1:00 rest		6 Squats (p. 114)		6 Lunges each side (p. 140)
10 Marching Twists (p. 133)		10 Supermans (p. 136)		12 Mason Twists (p. 138)		6 Push-Ups (p. 113)
5 Push-Ups (p. 113)	rest	5 Lunges each side (p. 140)	rest	12 Marching Twists (p. 133)	rest	8 Squats (p. 114)
1:00 rest		10 Bird Dogs (p. 136)		1:00 rest		1:00 rest
1:00 Walk		10 Wood Chops (p. 137)		:35 Jog		:40 Jog
:30 Jog		1:00 rest		:45 Walk		:40 Walk
1:00 Walk		:35 Jog		:35 Jog		:40 Jog
:30 Jog		:45 Walk		:45 Walk		:40 Walk
1:00 Walk		:35 Jog		:35 Jog		:40 Jog
--		:45 Walk		:45 Walk		:40 Walk
--		:35 Jog		--		--
--		:45 Walk		--		--

Prep Program *week 2*

Note: Rest and recovery are vital to the success of the program and should be included as prescribed on the schedule.

MON	TUE	WED	THU	FRI	SAT	SUN
rest	:45 Jog	rest	:45 Jog	rest	1:00 Jog	retake Initial Test (p. 113)
	:45 Walk		:30 Walk		1:00 Walk	
	:45 Jog		:45 Jog		:45 Jog	
	:45 Walk		:30 Walk		:45 Walk	
	:45 Jog		:45 Jog		1:00 Jog	
	:45 Walk		:30 Walk		:30 Walk	
	14 Wood Chops (p. 137)		10 Squats (p. 114)		16 Wood Chops (p. 137)	
	7 Lunges each side (p. 140)		8 Push-Ups (p. 113)		14 Hip Raises (p. 134)	
	10 Supermans (p. 136)		12 Bird Dogs (p. 136)		8 Push-ups (p. 113)	
	12 Hip Raises (p. 134)		12 Mason Twists (p. 138)		10 Lunges each side (p. 140)	
	:45 Jog		1:00 Jog		:45 Jog	
	:45 Walk		1:00 rest		:30 Walk	
	:45 Jog		1:00 Jog		1:00 Jog	
	:45 Walk		1:00 rest		:30 Walk	
	:45 Jog		--		1:00 Jog	
	:45 Walk		--		1:00 Walk	

Domination Level Alpha: 3-Week Race-Day-Ready Program

Looking for a beginner level? Not here. I chose to call it "Domination Level Alpha"; you deserved an audacious title to match your amazing new goals. This program is designed for those who are relatively new to fitness or coming back from taking some time off from athletic activities. Whether this is your first or fifth mud run, if you're able to complete the initial test in 35 to 40 minutes, this is the right place to start.

Domination Level Alpha will get you ready for an event that's about 24 days away. Your body needs the extra few days for rest and recovery before you tackle the course. Before you jump right in, you need to familiarize yourself with the functional cross-training exercises: pushing, pulling, and lifting for the Strength Workout and an over, under, across, and through routine for the Dexterity Workout. Starting on Day 3, we add some additional running to the mix.

Domination Level Alpha is performed three times per week with at least one day of rest between workouts. This is a wraparound-style program, so you'll be alternating workouts and rest days for the entire three weeks.

PROGRAM GUIDELINES

The results you'll get from the Strength and Dexterity workouts are directly proportional to the intensity you put into them–you choose the weight, speed, and tenacity for each rep based on your ability and your goals. You're the one putting the weight into the bucket or choosing which rock or log to use.

For example: "50-Yard Sandbag Carry" can be performed as:

- Walking 50 yards with one, two, or even three sandbags
- Jogging or sprinting 50 yards with a sandbag
- Progressing 50 yards out, 50 yards back
- Lifting and pressing the sandbag with each step
- Lunges, crawling, etc.

It's up to you how you execute—get it?

Perform each exercise in the set with little to no rest in between. Beginners, please rest and hydrate as needed. If you feel lightheaded or dizzy, stop exercising immediately. Seek medical help if condition persists after resting or you feel any sharp pains or blurriness of vision.

Start each training session with a 3- to 5-minute warm-up, and end the workout with at least 5 minutes of stretching (starting on page 142).

TESTING YOUR PROGRESS

How was your time? Have you improved significantly since you took that same test three weeks ago? If you followed the program and put the hard work and effort in, I'm extremely confident that you have. If not, it's probably a good idea for you to work through the Domination Level Alpha program again, this time with a higher level of intensity. No one said it was going to be easy, so keep it up and you'll see a marked improvement! Don't worry, the 5-week CRUSH IT Program will be ready whenever you are.

Domination Level Alpha Program *week 1*

Note: Rest and recovery are vital to the success of the program and should be included as prescribed on the schedule.

MON	TUE	WED	THU	FRI	SAT	SUN
Strength Workout (p. 81)	rest	Dexterity Workout (p. 101)	rest	Strength Workout (p. 81)	rest	Dexterity Workout (p. 101)
				2:00 rest		2:00 rest
				5:00 easy jog warm-up		2-mile easy jog
				10:00 moderate run		
				5:00 easy jog cool-down		

Domination Level Alpha Program *week 2*

Note: Rest and recovery are vital to the success of the program and should be included as prescribed on the schedule.

MON	TUE	WED	THU	FRI	SAT	SUN
rest	Strength Workout (p. 81)	rest	Dexterity Workout (p. 101)	rest	Strength Workout (p. 81)	rest
	2:00 rest		2:00 rest		2:00 rest	
	1-mile easy jog warm-up		2-mile easy jog cool-down		2-mile moderate run	
	1-mile moderate run				1-mile easy jog cool-down	
	1-mile easy jog cool-down					

Domination Level Alpha Program   *week 3*

Note: Rest and recovery are vital to the success of the program and should be included as prescribed on the schedule.

MON	TUE	WED	THU	FRI	SAT	SUN
Sets 1 and 2 from Strength Workout (p. 81)		Strength Workout (p. 81)		Dexterity Workout (p. 101)		retake the Initial Test (timed)
2:00 rest		2:00 rest		2:00 rest		5 Push-Ups (p. 113)
	rest	1-mile easy warm-up jog	rest	1-mile moderate run	rest	5 Squats (p. 114)
				2-mile easy jog		
Sets 1 and 2 from Dexterity Workout (p. 101)		1-mile moderate run		1-mile moderate run		1-mile run
		1-mile easy jog		1-mile easy jog		rest as needed, repeat twice (3 rounds total)

The CRUSH IT Program

Well, hello there, Speedy! Welcome to your own personal little guide to dominate each obstacle, smoke other competitors, and crush the most bad-ass courses on the planet. If you picked up this book to get faster and stronger, you've made it to the section that you've been dreaming of. The 5-week CRUSH IT Program is designed to make you cry for mercy and then beg for more. Buckle up, here we go!

Before you get started, you need to familiarize yourself with the functional cross-training exercises I described in "Prepare to Dominate All Obstacles" (page 69). I've developed three different workouts to get you ready for race day: Strength Workout—Pushing, Pulling & Lifting Stuff; Dexterity Workout—Over, Under, Across & Through Stuff; Speed & Endurance Workout—Torch the Course.

The CRUSH IT Program is performed every other day, sometimes two workouts in one day. No one ever said it'd be easy. It'll challenge you and make you stronger and faster and increase your endurance. I'm guessing you'll enjoy it a little bit, too. Below is an example of a wrap-around workout schedule starting on a Monday.

Monday: Workout
Tuesday: Rest
Wednesday: Workout
Thursday: Rest
Friday: Workout
Saturday: Rest
Sunday: Workout
Monday: Rest

PROGRAM GUIDELINES

The results you'll get from the workouts are directly proportional to the intensity you put into them—you choose the weight, speed, and tenacity for each rep based on your ability and goals. You're the one putting the weight into the bucket, choosing which rock or log to use, and deciding how hard you're going to sprint. If you feel the workout is too easy, you're not pushing hard enough or need a heavier object.

For example: "50-Yard Sandbag Carry" can be performed as:

- Walking 50 yards with one, two, or even three sandbags
- Jogging or sprinting 50 yards with a sandbag
- Progressing 50 yards out, 50 yards back
- Lifting and pressing the sandbag with each step
- Lunges, crawling, etc.

It's up to you how you execute—get it?

Perform each exercise in the set with little to no rest in between. If you're new to strenuous workouts, are you sure you're in the right place? Always remember to rest and hydrate as needed. If you feel lightheaded or dizzy, stop exercising immediately. Seek medical help if condition persists after resting or you feel any sharp pains or blurriness of vision.

Start each training session with a 3- to 5-minute warm-up, and end the workout with at least 5 minutes of stretching (starting on page 142).

Completing the CRUSH IT Program once doesn't necessarily mean you're as strong, fast, and dexterous as you can possibly be. Use this program between events and raise the intensity, reps, or weights as needed to get the results you want!

The CRUSH IT Program   *week 1*

Note: Rest and recovery are vital to the success of the program and should be included as prescribed on the schedule.

MON	TUE	WED	THU	FRI	SAT	SUN
Strength Workout (p. 81)		Dexterity Workout (p. 101)				Strength Workout (p. 81)
						2:00 rest
2:00 rest		2:00 rest		Speed & Endurance Workout (p. 108)		1-mile moderate run
	rest		rest		rest	10 Burpees (p. 139)
3-mile jog		1-mile weighted backpack walk (p. 140)				repeat run & Burpees twice (3 total rounds)

The CRUSH IT Program   *week 2*

Note: Rest and recovery are vital to the success of the program and should be included as prescribed on the schedule.

MON	TUE	WED	THU	FRI	SAT	SUN
			Speed & Endurance Workout (p. 108)		Dexterity Workout (p. 101)	
	Morning: Strength Workout (p. 81)				2:00 rest	
			2:00 rest		.5-mile weighted backpack walk, brisk pace (p. 140)	
rest		rest		rest	20 Squats (p. 114)	rest
	Evening: Dexterity Workout (p. 101)		50 Burpees (rest as needed) (p. 139)		.5-mile weighted backpack walk, brisk pace (p. 140)	
					20 Squats (p. 114)	

The CRUSH IT Program *week 3*

Note: Rest and recovery are vital to the success of the program and should be included as prescribed on the schedule.

MON	TUE	WED	THU	FRI	SAT	SUN
Morning: 1:00 sprint + 1:00 rest; repeat (10) total reps	rest	Speed & Endurance Workout (p. 108)	rest	*Morning:* Strength Workout (p. 81)	rest	Speed & Endurance Workout (p. 108)
		2:00 rest				
		22 Burpees (p. 139)				
Evening: Strength Workout (p. 81)		2:00 rest		*Evening:* Strength Workout (p. 81)		
		22 Burpees (p. 139)				

The CRUSH IT Program *week 4*

Note: Rest and recovery are vital to the success of the program and should be included as prescribed on the schedule.

MON	TUE	WED	THU	FRI	SAT	SUN
rest	Strength Workout (p. 81)	rest	Strength Workout (p. 81)	rest	Speed & Endurance Workout (p. 108)	rest
	2:00 rest		2:00 rest		2:00 rest	
	1:00 sprint + 1:00 rest; repeat (5) total reps		.5-mile Weighted Backpack Walk at brisk pace (p. 140)		40 Burpees (p. 139)	
			20 squats		2:00 rest	
			.5-mile Weighted Backpack Walk at brisk pace (p. 140)		40 Burpees (p. 139)	
			22 Lunges (p. 140)			

The CRUSH IT Program   *week 5*

Note: Rest and recovery are vital to the success of the program and should be included as prescribed on the schedule.

MON	TUE	WED	THU	FRI	SAT	SUN
Morning: 1:00 sprint + 1:00 rest; repeat (10) total reps	rest	*Morning:* Strength Workout (p. 81)	rest	Speed & Endurance Workout at easy pace (p. 108)	rest	repeat Initial Test (Timed) (p. 113)
Evening: Strength Workout (p. 81)		*Evening:* Dexterity Workout (p. 101)				2:00 rest
						45 Burpees (p. 139)

Training Grounds

Prior to your first obstacle race, when did you have the opportunity to scale an 8-foot wall? Jump over and under obstacles that were made to get your nose down in the dirt? Was the last time you saw a climbing rope in middle school? How about climbing a cargo net while suspended by a harness 50 feet in the air?

Well, now you can head to dedicated training and adventure facilities and practice some of the techniques that you've learned in this book and also notch some incredible once-in-a-lifetime thrills!

VictoryQuest

Obstacle Race Training Facility & Event Location, Lincoln, NE

Launched: *2012*

Course Distance: *5K–10K (depending on configuration)*

Obstacles: *25+ fixed and moveable obstacles*

Terrain: *Mostly flat with elevation changes around natural features*

Signature Obstacle: *The Immense Fence*

Hardest Obstacle: *The Kill Box*

Gear/Clothing: *Comfortable, exercise clothes that you don't mind getting dirty. During training, you can skip the muddy sections and focus on developing your skills on specific obstacles. Closed-toe shoes are required; gloves may be useful for rope-based obstacles and a hindrance for Immense Fence and others.*

Atmosphere: *Extremely family-friendly, this challenging course was created by two families and welcomes adventurers of all ages.*

VictoryQuest is a fixed-location obstacle race training center and event venue located smack-dab in the middle of the USA. At their hundred-acre facility you can tackle a 5K-plus course featuring climbing walls from 5- to 8-feet tall, jump, climb, crawl, and scurry over and under obstacles of all shapes and sizes or in and out of mud pits, scamper over a fallen tree across a stream, or navigate your way over 30 feet of massive hay bales in a family-friendly atmosphere that draws from the local community as well as adventure racers from all over the world. Inspired, creative obstacles abound: Hadrian's Wall is one of the most unique climbing walls, featuring a dozen vertical tires lashed together with over 600 feet of rope;

the Immense Fence is a challenging double-billboard-design horizontal climbing wall with a hand-over-hand pipe transition in the middle.

Their 15,000-square-foot indoor training facility has over 50 yards of obstacles where your feet never touch the ground. Like no other gym in the world, this subterranean playground of pain has you climbing, swinging, gripping, and jumping over a dozen different obstacles, all the while strengthening your upper body and preparing you for any obstacle you'll face during a race.

VictoryQuest is available year-round for individual and group training, corporate retreats, and team building, as well as hosting events organized by third parties.

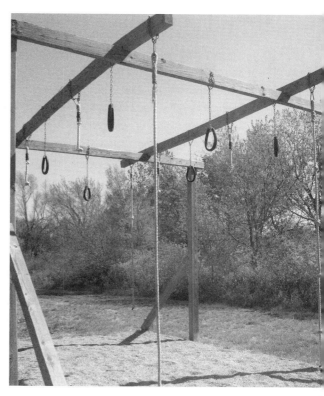

Flagstaff Extreme

Tree-top Obstacle Course, Flagstaff, AZ

Launched: 2012

Course Distance: Kid's course and 4 adult courses of varying distances

Obstacles: 72 elements to navigate, 6 zip lines

Terrain: 20–60' off the ground, suspended in trees

Signature Obstacle: Tarzan ropes, where Flagstaff Extremers have to hang on, just like Tarzan, and swing from one tree to the next to continue with the course; Tarzan calls are encouraged

Hardest Obstacle: All elements of the Black Course

Gear/Clothing: Course is at over 7,000 feet in elevation—wear temperature-appropriate clothing; safety harnesses are provided, fingerless gloves are recommended. Do not wear open-toed shoes, flip-flops, slip-on shoes, loose baggy clothing, or shirts wrapped around the waist; long hair must be tied back and eyeglasses must be secured. No jewelry (especially necklaces or loose bracelets that could get caught in equipment) is recommended.

Special Considerations: Make sure you're hydrated, nourished, and acclimated to the elevation; individuals will fatigue faster at 7,000 feet than at sea level.

No mud, no gladiators, no used tires to run through or barbed wire to crawl under—Flagstaff Extreme is a treetop adventure course that contains a series of exciting physical challenges suspended in trees at various heights. The park consists of 72 aerial challenges including cable bridges, Tarzan ropes, zip lines, swings, ladders, and other elements divided into four color-coded courses for juniors, adults, and kids. Safety is always first: participants of all ages are secured to a lifeline and wear a harness so that they can experience new thrills and test personal limits in a controlled environment.

Each course will challenge you mentally as it's up to you to figure out and navigate each obstacle. Making decisions 60 feet up in the air is a lot harder than you may think! As for the physical challenge, each course gets progressively more difficult in terms of the complexity and challenge of surprises that face each adventurer. While the courses can be completed by most individuals, tackling each successive course is a lot of work that will test your core, legs, and arms.

Flagstaff Extreme is a full-body, functional workout at its best, and ropes, climbing walls, swings, cargo nets, and even a suspended skateboard are all part of the course.

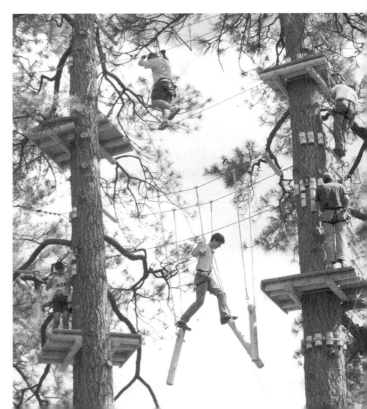

Getting Ready to Race

OK, you've completed all the physical training to get your body ready to crush any course and learned the proper techniques to conquer any obstacles. You've steeled your mind to vanquish any fear or trepidation, leaving no lingering doubts that you can reach your goals on race day. With less than a week before the big day, what else do you have to do? Prepare and test your gear!

In the "Gear Guide" on page 26, we covered shoes, clothes, gloves, and any miscellaneous stuff (like earplugs and gaiters) that you may wear on race day. A week before your race, pick out exactly what you plan on wearing. If you're missing anything or have anything new that you want to buy, get it now. Don't wait until the night before the race to go shopping, and absolutely don't break in new shoes during a race (or be prepared for a visit from the blister fairy)!

FIVE TO SEVEN DAYS BEFORE THE RACE, PERFORM THE FOLLOWING ROUTINE

Wake up at the same time you'd be getting up for your race; include the commute.

Eat the exact same meal you would on race morning; it should be hearty enough to give you the energy you need while not being too heavy on your stomach. You may need to do some research and testing to find your perfect balance during your training. I learned my pre-race meal from my *7 Weeks to a Triathlon* coauthor and professional triathlete, Lewis Elliot: steel-cut oatmeal with cinnamon, a whole banana, and a couple cups of black coffee.

Get all your gear on, from shoes to clothes and even earplugs and elbow sleeves. The goal is to test your race gear under race conditions. If you don't put it on, you won't know!

Go for a 1-mile jog/run, approximately at what you plan your race pace to be. If you've progressed all the way through the CRUSH IT Program, you should have a solid idea about proper pacing, and this should just be a warm-up. Leave your cell phone or iPod home because it's about to get more exciting…

Get wet—100% soaked. Go jump in a lake or pool; drag out the garden hose and make sure every last bit of your clothing and body is drenched. The colder the water, the better. If you have the *cojones*, take an ice bath. It'll only help you prepare for the frigid horrors you may see on race day!

Army crawl on your elbows and knees for 20 yards, turn around, and bear crawl back to your starting position. Pick an area that matches course terrain; you should be good and dirty.

Go for a 2-mile run, this time picking out stuff to climb on top of, scurry under, crawl through, or jump over. If you followed the fitness programs, you should already know the moves and have located what things you need near your neighborhood. If not, pick stuff that you won't break and/or hurt yourself in the process. Conquer your chosen obstacles, and run back home.

Did anything fall off? Get any chafing? Blisters? Did your gloves get too slippery to grab or pull yourself over things? Now's the time to figure it out and make the necessary changes and adjustments. Test again if necessary, making sure your clothes have time to be cleaned and dried before the race.

> **TIP:** Here's one tip that'll help you prepare for the icy plunge that a lot of events feature: The week before the race, take the coldest shower you possibly can every day. That's it. If you can handle a really cold shower for a few minutes, then you can brave a 30-second dip in an ice bath on race day.

RACE-DAY MORNING   I'm not trying to sound like your mom, but even just a little preparation goes a long way. The night before, make sure you know how to get to the race, how long it'll take, the price of parking, how early you need to show up to get checked in and sign your waiver before your heat starts, and all the other little things (like whether they have a bag drop and showers afterward).

Pack a change of clothes (including shoes or flip-flops for the drive home), a towel, and something small to munch on (like a granola bar) if you have a long drive and need a little more nutrition pre-race. Baby wipes are great to get some extra grime off, and cotton swabs and saline solution help cleaning out ears and eyes of muck. Unless you're a big fan of port-o-johns, wake up a little earlier and take care of your bathroom visit before you leave the house if you can. Apply sport sunscreen before you get dressed, so you cover any of the areas that may get exposed when you're out on the course.

At the event, leave anything that you don't want to get muddy, broken, or lost in your car from the get go. It may be your intention to go register and come back to the car to drop off your priceless heirloom eye patch, but stuff happens and you might forget. If you leave your smartphone in your pocket during a race, it'll most likely end up pretty dumb, the same as you'll feel. Apply another round of sunscreen when you get out of the car, especially if it has been more than an hour and a half since you left home. Don't leave valuables in your race drop bag; the race staff isn't responsible for it and you don't need that headache. The only things I recommend in that bag are a change of clothes, a towel, and a back-up car key on a key ring, clipped to the belt loop of the shorts in the bag. I'm not going to tell you where to "hide" your keys on your vehicle, but there are at least 11 decent spots where you can place your keys so you can access them from the outside after the race. Inside bumpers, on top of tires, and inside the fuel door all make sense, but I'm not responsible if your car gets jacked.

Take care of your registration and waiver signing first, then walk around the expo or spectate. Some races may even let you choose an earlier heat if you show up before your appointed time. Check out the course as much as you can; some may confuse scouting with cheating, but I say if it's visible then watch some other competitors tackle it for some great tips. Re-check your gear and attire, make sure you're hydrated, and jog around a bit about 10–15 minutes before your anticipated start to warm up. Head over to the corral when the announcer greets your wave.

Position yourself in the starting corral based on your goals. If you're looking to dominate the course and climb the winner's podium, march right up front and claim your spot. First-timers should make way for more experienced or faster-looking runners (although you never can tell if that couple in the Ninja Turtles outfits are really world-class athletes) so they don't get trampled once the gun goes off. Be responsible and realistic in your athletic ability; while you have as much right to the course as any other paying competitor, you don't want to be the one causing a traffic jam holding up other racers at an obstacle, do you?

Take a deep breath and remember all the training you've done to prepare; the race will be challenging, but you're ready to crush it! When the starter's gun goes off, keep your excitement in check and take a moderate pace; you don't want to burn yourself out immediately. When you're moving over, under, around, and through each obstacle, try to keep the same relative level of exertion so you don't drain all your energy by sprinting the intervals between obstacles. Attack the course, but do it wisely and within your ability so you can stay strong all the way to the finish!

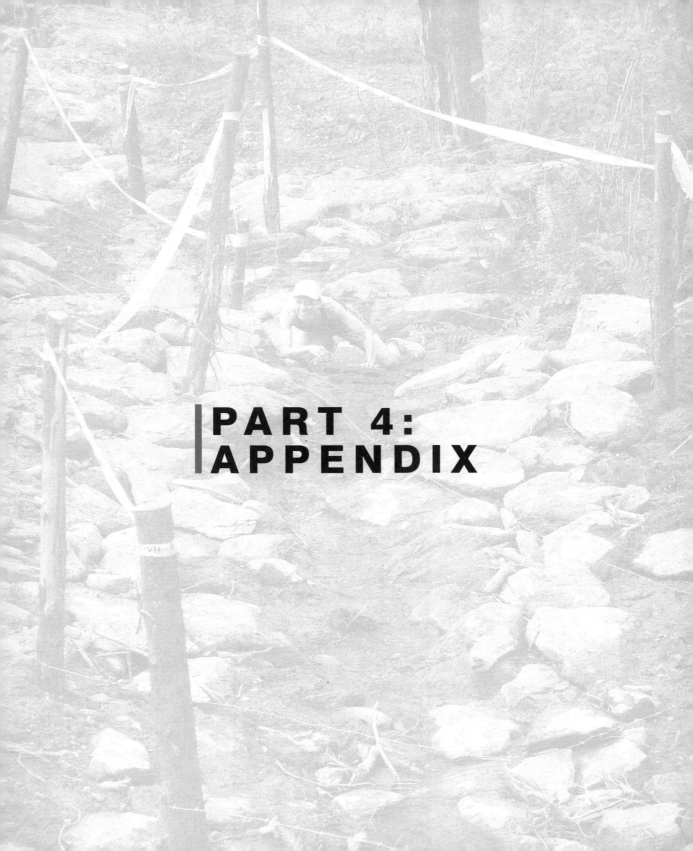

PART 4:
APPENDIX

Prep Program Exercises

Marching Twist

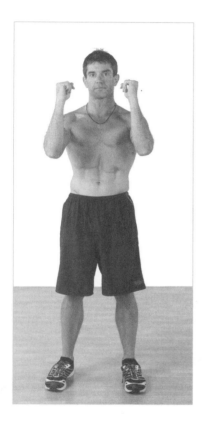 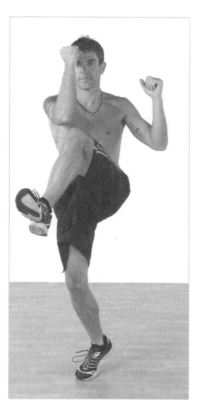 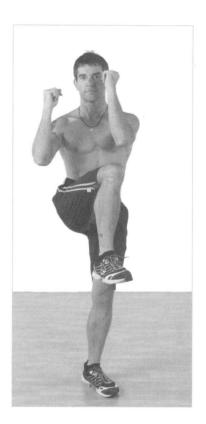

1 Stand tall with your feet shoulder-width apart. Bring your arms in front of you and bend your elbows 90 degrees.

2 Twist your torso to the right and raise your left knee to your right elbow.

3 Repeat with your right knee and left elbow. A little hop with the bottom foot helps you keep your momentum going from leg to leg.

Hip Raise

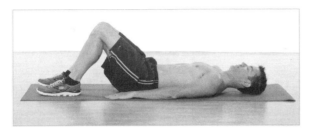 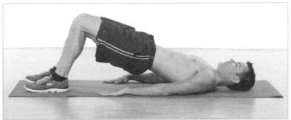

1 Lie on your back with your knees bent and feet flat on the floor, as close to your butt as possible. Extend your hands toward your hips and place your arms and palms flat on the floor at your sides.

2 Engage your abdominal muscles to keep your core tight, and exhale while you press your feet into the floor and raise your hips and lower back up, forming a straight line from your sternum to your knees. Do not push your hips too high or arch your back. Hold this position for 3 to 5 seconds, and then inhale and slowly return to starting position.

That's 1 rep.

Push-Up

1 Place your hands on the ground approximately shoulder-width apart, making sure your fingers point straight ahead and your arms are straight but your elbows not locked. Step your feet back until your body forms a straight line from head to feet. Your feet should be about 6 inches apart with the weight in the balls of your feet. Engage your core to keep your spine from sagging; don't sink into your shoulders.

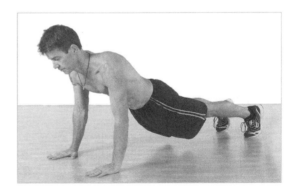

2 Inhale as you lower your torso to the ground and focus on keeping your elbows as close to your sides as possible, stopping when your elbows are at a 90-degree angle or your chest is 1 to 2 inches from the floor.

Using your shoulders, chest, and triceps, exhale and push your torso back up to starting position.

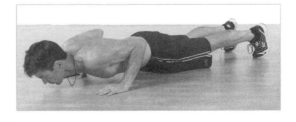

Squat

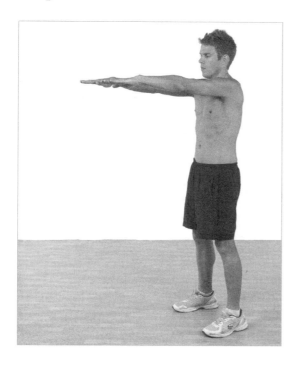

1 Stand tall with your feet shoulder-width apart and toes pointed slightly outward, about 11 and 1 o'clock. Raise your arms until they're parallel to the floor.

2 Bend at the hips and knees and "sit back" just a little bit as if you were about to sit directly down into a chair. Keep your head up, eyes forward, and arms out in front of you for balance. As you descend, contract your glutes while your body leans forward slightly so that your shoulders are almost in line with your knees. Your knees should not extend past your toes and your weight should remain between the heel and the middle of your feet—do not roll up on the balls of your feet. Stop when your knees are at 90 degrees and your thighs are parallel to the floor. If you feel your weight is on your toes or heels, adjust your posture and balance until your weight is in the middle of your feet.

Push straight up from your heels back to starting position. Don't lock your knees at the top of the exercise. That's 1 rep.

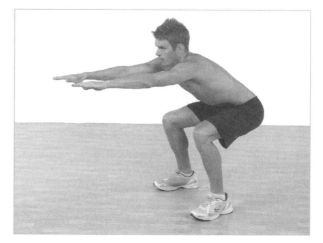

Superman

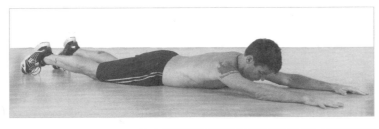

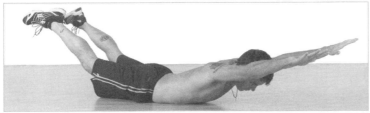

1 Lying face down on your stomach, extend your arms directly out in front of you and your legs behind you. Keep your knees straight as if you were flying.

2 In a slow and controlled manner, contract your erector spinae and raise your arms and legs about 6 to 8 inches off the floor. Hold for 5 seconds.

Lower slowly back to starting position.

Bird Dog

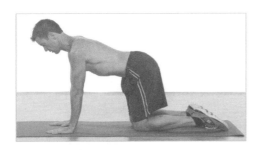

1 Get on your hands and knees with your legs bent 90 degrees, knees under your hips, toes on the floor, and your hands on the floor directly below your shoulders. Keep your head and spine neutral; do not let your head lift or sag. Contract your abdominal muscles to prevent your back from sagging; keep your back flat from shoulders to butt for the entire exercise.

2 In one slow and controlled motion, simultaneously raise your right leg and left arm until they're on the same flat plane as your back. Your leg should be parallel to the ground, not raised above your hip; your arm should extend directly out from your shoulder and your biceps should be level with your ear. Hold this position for 3 to 5 seconds and then slowly lower your arm and leg back to starting position.

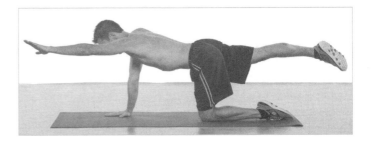

That's 1 rep. Switch sides and repeat.

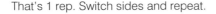

Wood Chop

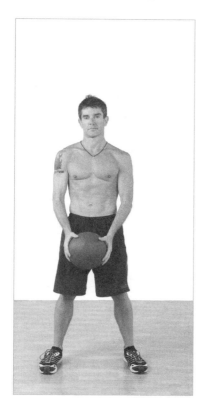 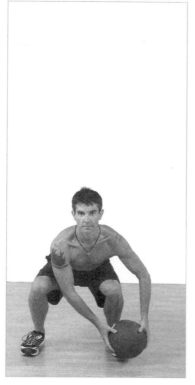 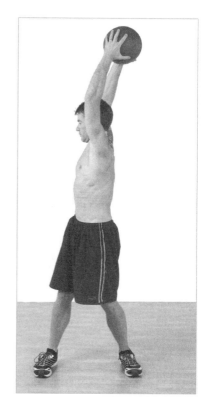

1 Stand tall with your feet shoulder-width apart, holding a medicine ball in front of you.

2 Lower your body into a squat until your knees are bent 90 degrees and bring the ball down to touch your left foot.

3 Stand tall, twisting your torso to the right and lifting your arms straight up over your head. Your left shoulder should be in front and you should be looking to the right.

Repeat to the other side.

Mason Twist

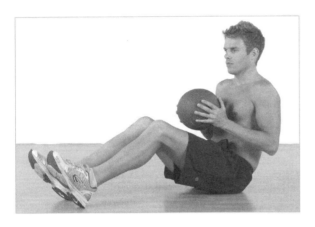

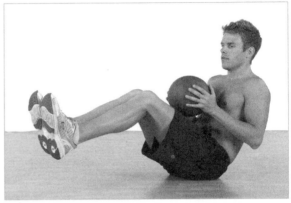

1 Sit on the floor with your knees comfortably bent, feet on the floor, arms bent 90 degrees, and hands holding a medicine ball or weight in front of your chest.

2 Lift your feet about 4 to 6 inches off the floor and balance your body weight on your posterior. Keep your core tight to protect your back.

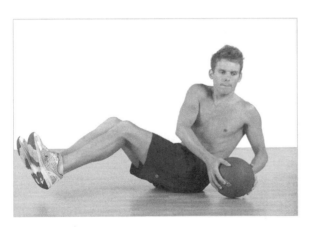

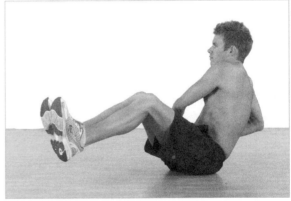

3 While maintaining the same hip position, twist your entire torso at the waist and touch the ball to the floor on the left side of your body.

4 Rotate back to center, keeping your feet off the floor and maintaining your balance using the supporting core muscles. Then rotate to your right and touch the ball to the floor.

Return to center. This is 1 rep.

CRUSH IT Program Exercises
Burpee

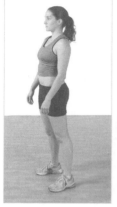

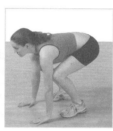

1 Stand tall with your back erect, feet shoulder-width apart, and toes rotated slightly outward.

2 Shift your hips backward and "sit back" for the squat, keeping your head up and bending your knees. Lean your weight forward and place your hands on the floor, inside, outside, or in front of your feet—whichever is more comfortable and gives you a nice, stable base.

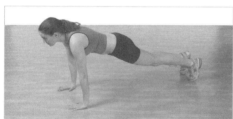

3 Kick your feet straight back so that you're now in a push-up starting position, forming a straight line from your head to your feet. Keep your core tight to maintain an erect spine.

4 Inhale as you lower your torso toward the floor for a push-up. Stop when your body is 1 to 2 inches from the floor.

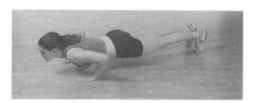

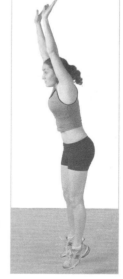

5 Exhaling, straighten your arms and propel your entire upper body off the floor while simultaneously bending your knees and bringing them toward your chest in order to plant your feet underneath you. You should end up back in the bottom position of a squat. Take a quick breath.

6 Swing your arms straight overhead, exhale, and push off from your feet to jump straight up in the air as high as possible. Land with your knees slightly bent to absorb the impact. That's 1 rep.

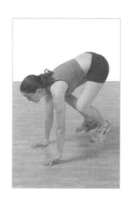

Forward Lunge

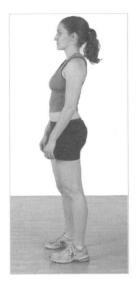
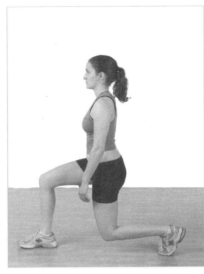

1 Stand tall with your feet shoulder-width apart and your arms hanging at your sides.

2 Take a large step forward with your right foot, bend both knees and drop your hips straight down until both knees are bent 90 degrees. Your left knee should almost be touching the ground and your left toes are on the ground behind you. Keep your core engaged and your back, neck, and hips straight at all times during this movement.

Pushing up with your right leg, straighten both knees and return to starting position. Repeat with the other leg.

Weighted Backpack Walk

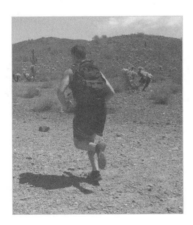

Throw some weight (books, rocks, a couple old laptops, or whatever you'd like) into a backpack and go for a nice, brisk walk. Keep your core engaged and your back straight; don't let the weight cause your posture to sag. Drive yourself forward with every step; this shouldn't be a walk in the park. Go ahead and find some hills and really kick this core, leg, and back workout up a notch.

Jumping Muscle-Up

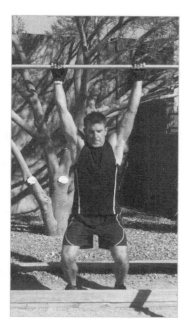

This is an advanced version of the Jumping Pull-Up (page 78). Pulling your chin up to a bar, door, or top of a wall is good, but getting your chest up that high is even better. This move takes a lot of strength and coordination to pull off, but don't get discouraged. Once you learn to explode upward and harness all your momentum to make the transition from pulling with your arms to pushing upward, you'll only get better. Keep trying; this is an important skill to master for scaling walls easily.

Performing a jumping muscle-up starts out just like the jumping pull-up: Stand below the bar, arms raised, hands open, bent at the waist, and knees slightly bent in a squat position. Forcefully jump straight up and grab the bar using every bit of momentum to pull your waist up to the bar. This will require an initial pull-up movement where you pull your body up using the large muscles of your upper back until the bar is just below your shoulders. When the bar reaches mid-chest, flare your elbows out on each side of your body and press your hands downward on the bar, extending your elbows to bring your waist up to the bar. Leaning your upper body slightly over the bar will help you extend your elbows and reach the top position of a jumping muscle-up.

Tip: Make sure your momentum is going straight up by standing about 6 inches back from directly under the bar; any swing forward with your legs below the bar will make it exponentially more difficult on your upper body to get you up over the top!

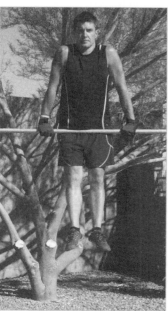

Warm-Ups & Stretches

Since you'll be pushing, pressing, and twisting your body during the workouts, it's very important to warm up before you stretch. Stretching prior to warming up can cause more damage than good to muscles, ligaments, and joints. When your muscles are cold, they're far less pliable and you don't receive any benefit from stretching prior to warming up. In this section are some dynamic warm-ups that'll get your heart rate up, loosen tight muscles, and prepare you for your workout.

After your workout, stretching will help you reduce soreness from the workout, increase range of motion and flexibility within a joint or muscle, and prepare your body for any future workouts. Stretching immediately post-exercise while your muscles are still warm allows your muscles to return to their full range of motion (which gives you more flexibility gains) and reduces the chance of injury or fatigue in the hours or days after an intense workout.

It's important to remember that even when you're warm and loose, you should never "bounce" during stretching. Keep your movements slow and controlled. The stretches in this section should be performed in order to optimize your recovery. Remember to exhale as you perform every deep stretch and rest 30 seconds in between each stretch.

Warm-Ups

Arm Circle

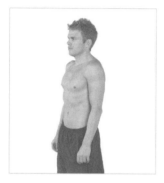 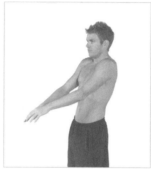 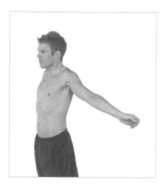

1 Stand with your feet shoulder-width apart.

2-3 Move both arms in a complete circle forward 5 times and then backward 5 times.

Lumber Jack

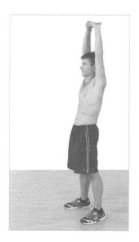 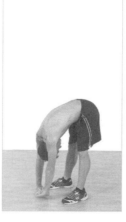

1 Stand with your feet shoulder-width apart and extend your hands overhead with elbows locked, fingers interlocked, and palms up.

2 Bend forward at the waist and try to put your hands on the ground (like you're chopping wood). Raise up and repeat.

Side Bend

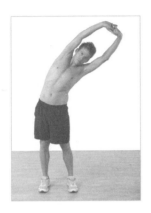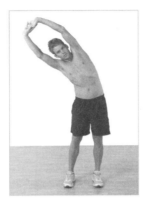

Stand with your feet shoulder-width apart and extend your hands overhead with elbows locked, fingers interlocked, and palms up. Bend side to side.

Around the World

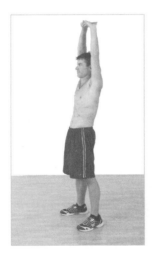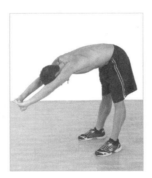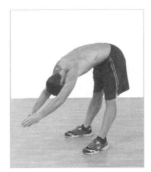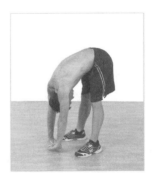

1 Stand with your feet shoulder-width apart and extend your hands overhead with elbows locked, fingers interlocked, and palms up. Keep your arms straight the entire time.

2–4 Bending at the hips, bring your hands down toward your right leg and in a continuous circular motion bring your hands toward your toes, then toward your left leg, and then return your hands overhead and bend backward.

Repeat three times, then change directions.

Stretches

Forearm & Wrist

Begin the stretch gently and allow your forearms to relax before stretching them to their full range of motion.

1 Stand with your feet shoulder-width apart and extend both arms straight out in front of you. Keep your back straight. Turn your right wrist to the sky and grasp your right fingers from below with your left hand. Slowly pull your fingers back toward your torso with your left hand; hold for 10 seconds.

2 Swap arms and repeat.

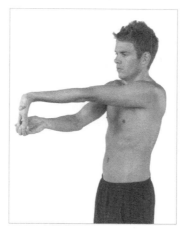 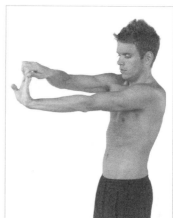

Shoulders

1 Stand with your feet shoulder-width apart and bring your left arm across your chest. Support your left elbow with the crook of your right arm by raising your right arm to 90 degrees. Gently pull your left arm to your chest while maintaining proper posture (straight back, wide shoulders). Don't round or hunch your shoulders. Hold your arm to your chest for 10 seconds.

2 Release and switch arms.

After you've done both sides, shake your hands out for 5 to 10 seconds.

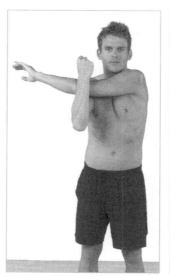 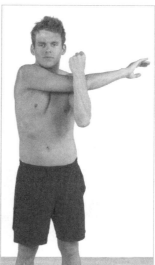

Shoulders & Upper Back

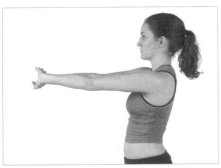

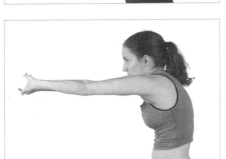

1 Stand with your feet shoulder-width apart and extend both arms straight out in front of you. Interlace your fingers and turn your palms to face away from your body. Keep your back straight.

2 Reach your palms away from your body. Exhale as you push your palms straight out from your body by pushing through your shoulders and upper back. Allow your neck to bend naturally as you round your upper back. Continue to reach your hands and stretch for 10 seconds.

Rest for 30 seconds then repeat. After you've done the second set, shake your arms out for 10 seconds to your sides to return blood to the fingers and forearm muscles.

Chest & Arms

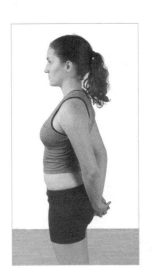

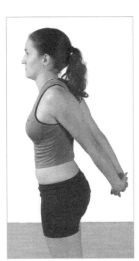

Clasp your hands together behind your lower back with palms facing each other. Keeping an erect posture and your arms as straight as possible, gently pull your arms away from your back, straight out behind you. Keep your shoulders down. Hold for 10 seconds.

Rest for 30 seconds and repeat.

Cobra

Lying on your stomach, place your hands directly under your shoulders with your fingers facing forward and straighten your legs and point your toes. Exhale and engage your core while lifting your chest off the floor and pushing your hips gently into the floor. Your arms help guide you through the movement, and your elbows should remain slightly bent at the top of the extension and your hips should remain in contact with the mat. Hold the up position for 15 to 30 seconds and then gently roll your upper body back to the floor. Hold for 30 seconds.

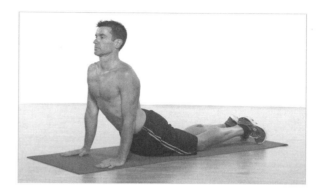

Child's Pose

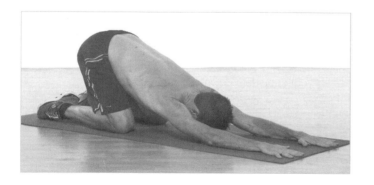

From a kneeling position, sit your buttocks back on your calves then lean forward and place your lower torso on your thighs. Extend your arms directly out in front of you, parallel to each other, and lower your chest toward the floor. Reach your arms as far forward as you can and rest your forearms and hands flat on the floor. Hold for 30 seconds.

Photo Credits

Index

Acknowledgments

There are so many people that made this book possible—it's impossible to thank them all. Selica, Joe, Andy, Richard, Carrie, and the entire team at Spartan Race embraced this project from the get-go and have been amazing to work with.

To Doug and Doug at VictoryQuest, Paul and the team at Flagstaff Extreme, Devon at Cahoots, Alex and Jane at Tough Mudder, Brad at Rugged Maniac, Lauren at Warrior Dash, Francis at LoziLu, Ashley at Run For Your Lives, Diane and Dave at Hero Rush, Mike and Carl at Obstacle Apocalypse, Rick at Scavenger Dash and Mad Mud Run, Gina and Keith at ROC Race and Del Mar Mud Run, Sam at Savage Race, Billy (Mr. Mouse) at Tough Guy, David and Shannon at Alpha Warrior, and Thomas at Bounce Boot Camp–your help, support, and enthusiasm have been absolutely invaluable. Thank you so much for providing the stories about your races and opening up your events for a behind-the-scenes peek!

Special thanks to Chris Lewis for being the brains and developer behind www.mudrunguide. com, and a huge thank you to my loving wife Kristen for putting up with my travel all over the country to check out cool events and spending every waking minute of 2012 talking/writing/ blogging/Facebooking about mud runs.

Contributors

The following individuals provided additional content:

Carrie Adams, Rad Racing and Spartan Chicked

Jonathan Nolan, Corn Fed Spartans

Devon Anderson, Cahoots Duo Challenge

Michael Sandercock, Obstacle Racers

Claire and Chris Treanor, CrossFit Blade, Phoenix, AZ

Some content was edited due to length. Please check out www.mudrunguide.com/fallenspartan to read the touching tribute Jonathan Nolan, Spartan Race, and the members of Corn Fed Spartans participated in to honor the memory of Steve Skidmore, a fellow obstacle racer who passed away during training.

About the Author

Brett Stewart is an endurance athlete and personal trainer residing in Phoenix, Arizona. An adrenaline junkie, Brett is an Ironman triathlete, ultramarathoner, and rabid obstacle racer. A proud father, husband, son, and brother, Brett has written numerous fitness books including *7 Weeks to a Triathlon*, *7 Weeks to Getting Ripped*, and *Ultimate Jump Rope Workouts*. He can be found online at www.7weekstofitness.com.

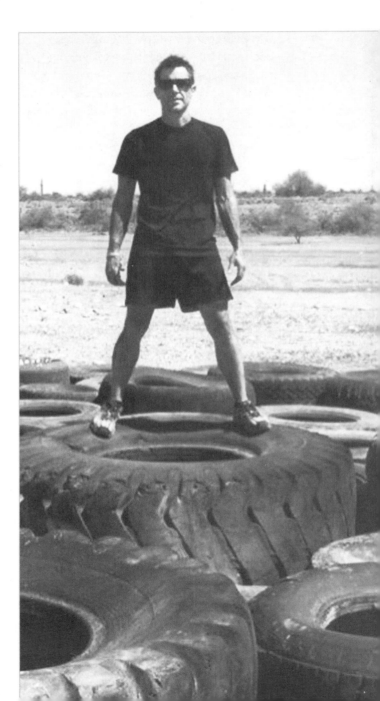